Runs in the Family

Raising Emotionally Healthy Children and Overcoming Mental Health Difficulties

By Jacqueline Campbell

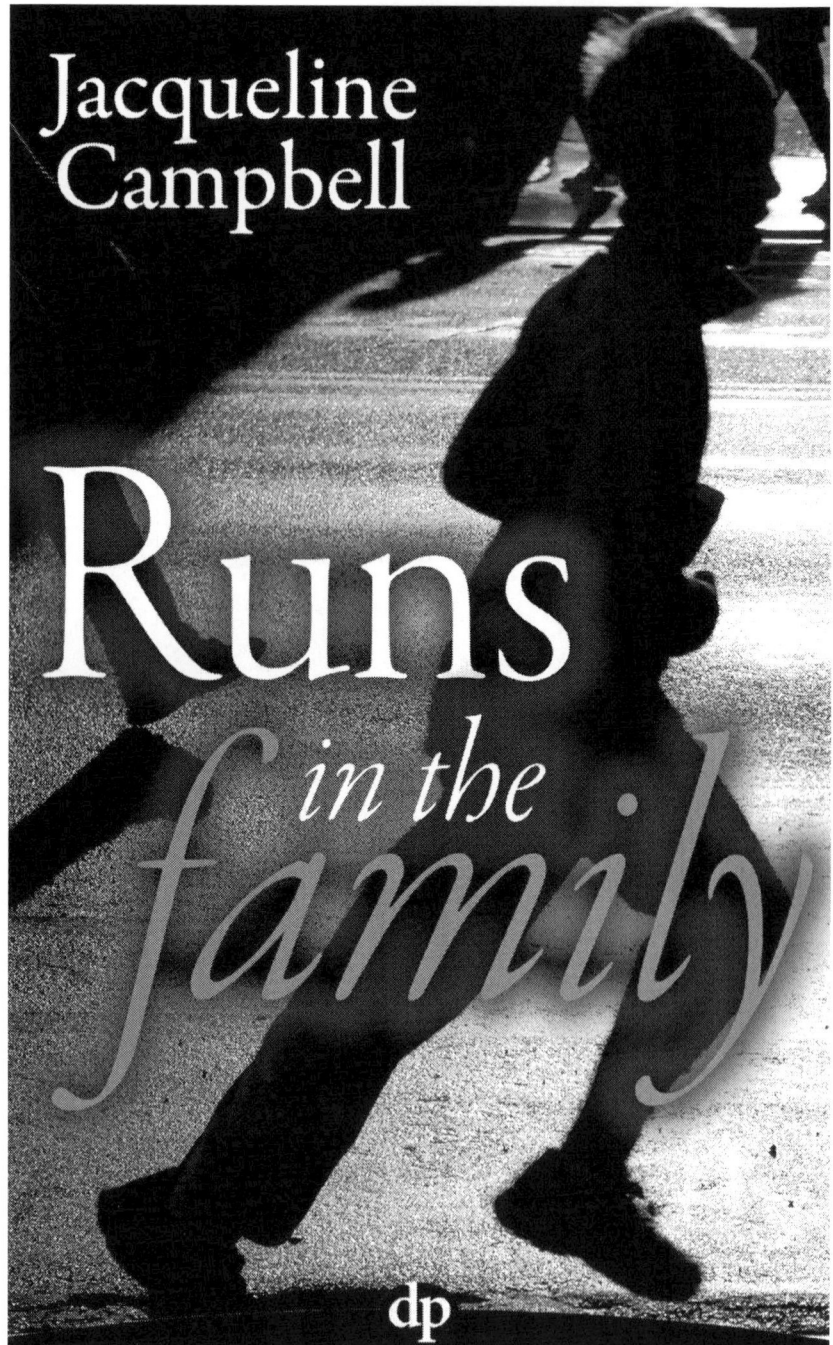

Jacqueline Campbell

Copyright © 2018 Jacqueline Campbell
All rights reserved. No part of this book may be reproduced in any form without permission in writing from the author. Reviewers may quote brief passages in reviews.
ISBN: 9781983232282
ISBN-1

Now I have a message
Now I want to create a movement
I have a reason bigger than life itself,
That reason for playing full-out to make a difference in the world through barriers that I believed I couldn't overcome, is my brother Julian
I live in the hope that this book will make him proud

FOREWORD

I'm very happy to be International Wellbeing Ambassador for Julian Campbell Foundation. I am pleased to be collaborating with Jacqueline the CEO of the foundation and have enjoyed spending time with young people promoting JCF's wellbeing movement on World Mental Health day 2017. I'm proud to be promoting an organisation that makes such a difference in the lives of young people.

I'm Toriano Jackson, although you may know me as Tito. When I was a teenager, my brothers and I, were blessed with international fame and success as The Jackson 5 after signing a record deal with Motown and releasing our debut single, I Want You Back. At 18 years old, I was married and a dad. I'm a proud and loving father of my sons, TJ, Taj and Taryll. Also, I'm proud to be a grandfather with all the privileges and blessings it brings. My sons are amazing and talented and wanting to be like their dad, formed 3T, a group promoted initially by my brother Michael. 3T found international success. Today, 50 years later, I'm still enjoying touring the world with my brothers Jackie, Marlon and Jemaine as the Jacksons and loving every minute.

Children are our future. Jacqueline's book, Runs in the Family is a great 'must have' for any parent or would be parent as it helps the reader form more loving relationships with their child. Also, through loving relationships, better communication stops barriers from growing which is really important for any young person's development. How else are we going to find out if their smile is really a smile or an upside-down frown?

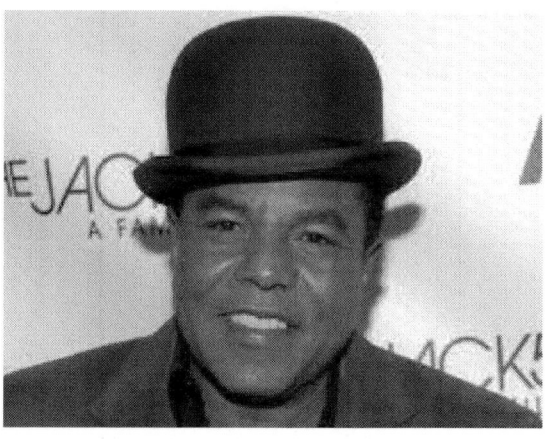

Tito Jackson – member of the Jackson 5

Also, you see that that your relationship with your child can teach you things about yourself that you never knew, so you're both learning! Through Runs in the Family, Jacqueline illustrates many examples from her own personal experiences and those from empowering and enabling young people through Julian Campbell Foundation. Her work is much needed and inspirational.

It is the fundamental right of every person and every child to be able to manage their own wellbeing especially in todays day and age where there are so many distractions and experiences that can bring on mental illness if it isn't managed when symptoms begin. We have to manage our wellbeing and make it a priority and Run's in the family benefits both the parent and the child to prosper and grow emotionally. I recommend that you read this book and pass it on to your friends and family when you've finished it to raise the profile of our wellbeing movement and the importance of wellbeing worldwide.

CONTENTS

Acknowledgements	ix
Introduction	Pg 1
Chapter 1 – The Big Solution Framework	Pg 7
Chapter 2 - The Big Solution Framework	Pg 17
Chapter 3 - What's the Point of Knowing How I Feel?	Pg 21
Chapter 4 - Rules for Peace and Harmony	Pg 36
Chapter 5 - Self-Care	Pg 43
Chapter 6 - What Are Your Key Actions to Avoid or Drop?	Pg 57
Chapter 7 - Keeping Your Word	Pg 67
Chapter 8 - Onward and Upward	Pg 74
Chapter 9 – Obstacles	Pg 84
Chapter 10 – Back to the Future	Pg 88
About the Author	Pg 90
Thank You	Pg 92

ACKNOWLEDGMENTS

This book idea came together through supporting many young people and their families and seeing that when parents and their children are supported individually, the children make the greatest progress in managing their moods and wellbeing.

First of all, I would like to thank God that I am where I am today and able to write something that, with His guidance, will make a real difference and impact in the lives of others and their families.

I want to acknowledge my mum and dad, my mother for showing me the importance of education in achieving my goals and my dad for showing me and teaching me the people skills to achieve them.

I want to acknowledge my friends Anne-Marie and Delia and my sister, Simone, for their support and encouragement through writing this book. Thanks to all the volunteers and supporters of the Julian Campbell Foundation, who, through their dedication and commitment, enabled our organisation to really make a difference with many young people and their families.

Thank you to all the children and young people that I have taught and supported over many years, as you have contributed to my life, my satisfaction that I have made a difference, and my enjoyment in seeing you achieve in your chosen careers.

Finally, thank you to the Difference Press, and to Maggie and Angela for their guidance, support and encouragement writing this book.

INTRODUCTION

Your child wasn't born with a manual. Come to think of it, neither were you. Didn't you wish that your parents understood you more? Even back then, everything was such a struggle! And these days, it's so much more complex to raise a child than ever before. Your child has to deal with situations and issues you may not have experienced yourself growing up: the strong pressure to achieve in school; being a victim or perpetrator of bullying; blended families; problems within peer groups at school; changing definitions of sexuality and confusion around them; the impact of cultural and social norms, including the increasing pressure from social media. Your child is justifiably overwhelmed.

You know mental health challenges are everywhere. You try not to worry too much, but still … you think about how you and family members have suffered, and about the fact that you have a close relative suffering from schizophrenia, bipolar disorder, depression … maybe someone in your family has even committed suicide. The thing is, no one has accepted that there's a problem, and everyone has carried on as if everything is ok, it's ok to hide whatever you're dealing with from everyone else. No one in your family has spoken about what happened, leaving you to deal with the bereavement and illness in your family alone. You've suffered through your own negative thoughts and depressive feelings about your family, about yourself, even some post-natal depression. Sure, things are slightly better now; your depression is mostly under control, but it's still easily triggered if you eat a lot of fast food and sweets, or drink a little too much alcohol.

Now that your second child is nine years old, you're beginning to feel really worried about his behaviour, and you suspect that he may have traits of depression himself. He's not as sociable as your first child, and he stays in his room for hours at a time. He's demanding and takes up a lot of your time; you are at your wits end. The really surprising thing is that his behaviour in school is completely different, and his teachers tell you that your son is an example to the others! He's intelligent and participates well in school, and everyone loves him. This makes you feel even more isolated, sure that your son's behaviour is your fault; you have your own struggles with depression, which you know is having an impact on your son. You doubt that you can give him the support he really needs.

You're afraid for his future, that if things are too difficult for your son, what seems like the beginning of depression may only get worse. What if he is struggling and feels unable to speak to anyone else in the family? You have an idea that it is really important to provide support for your son, maybe something artistic or creative to help him express himself, or a sport or other activity to promote a way that he can deal more positively with negative feelings. The attention that your son gets from you is, for the most part, negative attention; you feel like he doesn't listen to you and challenges everything you say. You are worn out and exhausted. You have stopped seeing your friends because you feel you can't tell them that although you love your son, you don't like him very much. You're afraid of being judged. It's all a struggle. When you go to the doctor, you don't feel really supported, and there are no community groups that you feel can guide you. You don't have peace of mind and are constantly questioning yourself. You feel completely lost.

You have been checking blogs and social media, searching for the nearest community groups so you can speak with them about your difficulties and get advice on how to provide support for your son. But in the meantime, you know that things will continue as they are, and you dread the thought that when your son gets into secondary school, the problem will get worse and more difficult for you to overcome. There'll be an impact on your love and the affinity between you and your son that can seem almost impossible to overcome. As he gets older, he'll probably blame you for that – and you worry that he'll be right to do so.

This book, *Runs in the Family*, will give you the tools to help you support your child as well as help you take powerful actions that will make a lasting difference for you, your family, and the way you live your life. By following each chapter, you will have an opportunity to work on and develop a different tool to further support both you and your child, giving you more peace of mind and a greater freedom and ease in the way you live your lives.

Instead of coping with your depression, you will see its importance in guiding you and showing you how to change your life and the life of your child for the better. This reflection in your life will give you greater clarity on how to continue forward with self-love, peace, patience, and structure. In place of confusion, there will be power, authority, and love between you and your child. Your relationship will positively impact the rest of your family. By using these tools to support your child, you will find the life of your dreams. Any period of emotional growth emerges from discomfort. We are moved to change, and we seek out new challenges as well as the tools to overcome them. When the challenges get bigger, we need new and improved tools to transcend them.

The bigger the challenge, the greater the opportunity for growth, giving us an invitation to step into our power and have the lives we dream of. Discomfort becomes its own tool; we don't stop until we find ourselves in a position that is comfortable enough to allow us to grow and develop. Author and spiritual teacher Marianne Williamson says it's our light we're afraid of, not our darkness, and that when we fill ourselves with light, it gives permission for everyone around us to do the same thing. It's the same for you. By allowing light into your life, you will have a positive impact on those around you, including your kids. You transform your relationships and your circumstances.

Of course we're full of fear. Fear is our way of staying safe and maintaining the status quo. Our fear believes it's trying to protect us from harm. Our hearts know that if we didn't take risks and try something different, our lives would be restricted and constrained and we wouldn't do anything. Caught between fear and heart, we stay stuck, hoping that each situation will resolve itself without us doing anything at all.

That is a dream. There's nothing wrong with dreams, they're important to keep us moving and achieving. However, it is your hope that you must listen to, as it is our hope (along with being uncomfortable in certain times of our lives) that guides us toward the solution. Fear will always be there, and it can be loud, so it is fear that we normally listen to. But when we give in to fear, we disempower ourselves from achieving our dreams.

So, acknowledge your fear. Thank it for its contribution. Listen to what your fear is telling you, in the same way you would listen to a friend's advice but probably decide not to take it. Start listening to your hope, and acknowledge your dreams instead. Fear tells you that it is impossible to have the life that you dream of, that it's normal not to have the perfect life, and that to try to do so is extremely dangerous and unrealistic. Hope tells you that you will have the life you dream of, and you will resolve those difficulties that are making you uncomfortable. Hope makes us look at whatever situation we're dealing with and gives us the strength to overcome everything, giving us new power and purpose in our lives.

This book will show you how to stop listening to your fears and start listening and taking action to achieve your hopes. In addition, you will remember dreams that you had long forgotten and thought were impossible to achieve. In this journey, you will look at yourself, your family, and your life in a totally different way, and accept yourself in a way that you have found difficult until now. Furthermore, your life will transform. Your emotional growth will surprise you, as well as how that growth comes to be reflected in the world around you.

You will see what's at the source of your emotions and why it's occurring as if you're a victim of your surroundings. You'll learn to start recognising your emotions, and see that your surroundings and environment are a reflection of those emotions. You'll see what it's like to be in your child's life, and feel what they're dealing with on a daily basis. You'll take action to eliminate three key behaviours that aren't working for you in your life and replace them with three, specific positive behaviours. Together, we will set up a structure that will foster emotional growth in your children and develop and a closeness and respect between you.

CHAPTER 1
What's the problem?

My Story

A lot of my life has revolved around mental health issues. I survived two assaults, and after turning to drugs to help take away the pain and the self-blame and self-loathing, I managed to deal with and overcome the feelings of depression, desperation, and sadness that had settled like a cloud over my head. My brother Julian had bipolar disorder, my mother chronic anxiety disorder, and my father depression. My brother was intelligent, talented, and a delight. He was far more intelligent than his years. When he was 11 years old and I was 13, I remember being very excited because I was going to the school disco for the first time in my life. My mum was only allowing me to go because my brother was coming, too. My brother's room was the only place that had a full-length mirror, and I wanted to check out my outfit and my hair. I rushed into his room only to be told, 'No! You can't come in yet, I'm doing electrolysis and collecting oxygen and hydrogen gas, you'll have to wait!'

'Electrolysis?' I thought. 'That's something that we do in school, not in our bedroom!' But this is how Julian was, always thinking about mixing chemicals together and making new things. When he was 14, he made a bomb that blew up the boys' cloakrooms at school. He was excluded for a few days. As Julian got older, he joined a gang, started drinking and taking drugs, and became ill. It took years to diagnose his bipolar disorder. We tried to support him all we could, but we really didn't know how to.

Finally, when my mum got so ill that she couldn't get to work, my brother went to a National Health Services (NHS) hospital for the first time. While in hospital, Julian was repeatedly assaulted, which understandably added to his depression. By this time, both my mum and dad were showing signs of being very ill. Dad was suffering from depression. Mum refused to accept that she was ill, and that stopped her from living the kind of life she really wanted. We couldn't support her because we didn't know what to do and we couldn't do better until we knew better. Because we didn't know how, her condition got worse over time.

Our family was divided. Some pointed fingers and judged us. Others were more sympathetic. Some weeks, I would see my mum's doctors, my brother's doctors, and my dad's doctors, listening to the advice of each doctor, asking questions about what we could do to help their progress, hoping that they would get better. My life was one challenge after another. There were always fights, arguments. It felt like I was firefighting all the time.

Somehow, I managed to continue my career as a consultant teacher and support my family with the help of a couple of really great cousins. Then, something really shocking and tragic happened. Julian had been sectioned for three months or so, being detained in hospital for assessment of his mental health and to get any treatment he might need. But just days after being discharged, my brother committed suicide on the day before his birthday. It was devastating and shocking. I was inconsolable, and from that moment, my life changed forever.

For the first few weeks after his death, I spent my time tracking Julian's every move before he'd killed himself. He'd gone to visit a few close friends and family members, me included, to say goodbye, but I didn't realise that I would be seeing him for the last time. After he died, I found a telephone message he'd left for me. I listened to this message several times a day, trying to get used to the fact that I would never hear his voice again. Part of me died inside. I struggled for the first two years without him in my life, finding the pain of his death difficult to bear and not knowing how to continue without him.

Then, two years after my brother's suicide, I found my purpose, and it came about because finally, I was the one who fell ill, at first with depression, and then with Chronic Fatigue Disorder or ME (Myalgic Encephalomyelitis). I had always taken my high energy for granted, and now, it had all disappeared.

The good thing about this was that I had to choose what I wanted to take forward in my life. I couldn't do everything I wanted to do, because my lack of energy really limited things. For this reason, I decided to focus on my charity work, as it really inspired me; I had already founded the Julian Campbell Foundation, and we were supporting children and families in our surrounding communities. We had trained up mentors in the community, and these mentors were supporting the young people who had undiagnosed stress, anxiety, and depression, helping them find ways of managing their wellbeing. We provided support and guidance for parents too, helping them to support their children and themselves emotionally.

In addition to focusing on this work, I decided to spend more time with my mum, to hang out with her and get to know her again. All those years of dedicating myself to my work had taken its toll on our relationship as a mother and daughter, and I had begun to see her and her illness as a burden, something I had to do. The love and affinity had gone. I realised that I didn't know who my mum was any more, and just saw her as a sick person needing help and support. Taking time with my mum was my opportunity to get behind her illness and understand the real reason for her condition. Through doing this, I fell in love with her again and saw just how delightful she is.

****

My career in education has been very successful. I have over 20 years of experience in education, and have taught science in some of the most difficult and challenging inner-city London schools. After getting excellent reviews as a teacher and manager of science from OFSTED, Office for Standards Education, Children's Services and Skills, I went into consultancy and used my knowledge to improve failing schools. I worked with many teachers and children with stress, anxiety, and depression, myself included.

I saw there was a need to support children and young people with depression as quite often, they're not shown how to manage their feelings and wellbeing when young. This is why, at the Julian Campbell Foundation, we support children and young people by showing them the skills they need to manage their wellbeing for life. Today, this is so important! Young people are dealing with exam stress, broken family living situations, confusion with their sexuality, bullying, social media, growing up and maturing, friendships and other relationships. In addition to this, it is common for young people to deal with bereavement, if not through the loss of their friends in schools (due to the knife crime epidemic in London), then through the loss of a loved one such as a parent or grandparent. It is not a common conversation to show someone how to deal with these powerful feelings. Because of this, 50 to 70 percent of adults who have mental illness had symptoms that showed up when they were children, but those symptoms were ignored, not spotted, or not dealt with very well.

If each child could identify their emotion and manage their feelings, therefore avoid stress, anxiety, or depression, can you imagine how powerful that could be for them for their lives? And when they grow into parenthood, these skills can be shown to their children.

I grew up being taught that education is most important. I'm not denying that it is. My education has enabled me to get countless jobs and promotions and make a difference that has been deep and lasting. I had no idea that the children who I first met when they were 10 years old would still be in my life in their twenties and thirties, that they would share their achievements and successes with me. This is a hidden advantage of teaching with my heart and soul, with a belief that you teach your students to have a better life and achieve better things than you have.

The Miracle of Life

Looking at my journey over the last 10 years, it is a miracle that I am still here! There were many times in the last decade when I didn't think I could get to where I am now, when I couldn't take another day of feeling the pain in my heart and soul. The pain of my brother dying was indescribable and like no other pain I'd ever felt before, completely unlike the trauma I'd experienced, for example, from physical assaults. My pain from being assaulted enabled me to continue (for a while) as if nothing had happened, largely because I smoked weed to numb the pain I was experiencing. The death of my brother was something on a totally different level. I didn't want to blot out anything or any emotions that I felt, as they were the only things I had linking me to him. I wanted to feel those emotions and love him with all my heart and soul. I remember the day of his funeral as clearly as if it were yesterday. It was the last time we were together in the same room before he was buried, my beautiful and talented brother.

I never thought I'd get used to the hurt and the pain that I had suffered. Neither could I ignore the feelings that were awakening a part of me that I didn't know. My old self died, the party lover who loved dancing through the night, and my new self, who wanted to change things and make a difference in the world, emerged. In a way, I was reborn, and through this miracle, I grew stronger and learned to love myself and life again. I have learned through tragedy that it is possible to reemerge like a chrysalis, a different creature, totally transformed.

Finding the Way

I figured it out by realising that I could not ignore my emotional or mental health. I was understandably focused on results and achievement (of myself, my students and the schools that I taught in), knowing that my most important job was telling the students that they could achieve whatever they wanted. But in focusing on helping others feel comfortable speaking about their health concerns and the things that were happening in their lives, I forgot about self-care. I just kept going until one day, I crashed due to ME, and my exhaustion simply couldn't be reversed, reduced, or eliminated by just a good night's sleep.

For all my life, I'd taken my copious amounts of energy for granted – until I couldn't even sit up in bed because it took too much energy to do that. I started listening to my body. I would rest for days (or sometimes weeks) at a time to store up energy in my body. I had no other choice – I was like a mobile phone that needed to top up its charge! Then I would have enough energy to do something that I wanted to do, but I had to be careful and not use too much energy. Walking about, for example, would deplete my stores of energy too quickly, and then I wouldn't be able to do what I wanted.

I started measuring my energy and emotional level at various times in the day and realised that every two weeks, I could go out and do something that I wanted to do, return home, and then, for the next few days, recharge. I started looking for foods that would increase my energy, such as proteins, and cut out my favourites: carbohydrates and chocolates. I stopped drinking alcohol and energy drinks for the same reason. Drinking an energy drink was like making a payment using a credit card … sooner or later, I'd have to pay it back. This would mean that shortly after the energy boost the energy drink gave me, I'd experience a massive slump.

Nowadays, I continue to monitor my energy and emotions to help me manage my wellbeing. In the case of mental health, it's as simple as being aware of my energy state and my emotional feelings: am I excited, calm, stressed, or feeling sad?

If I find myself becoming too stressed, for example, this would mean that I have high amounts of energy and negative emotions. In these moments, I know that I need to discharge or release some energy in a safe way, to stop me from burning out again with fatigue. I need to do something immediately to stop draining my energy and needlessly throwing it away.

What do I do to release stress? I go for a walk or a run. What do I do to improve my negative emotions? I go to church or I pray, speak with a good friend, listen to my favourite music – Michael Jackson or Amy Winehouse usually does it. All of these things will shift my mood state and give me back my power. All of this helps me to replenish my bucket of energy and stay in touch with my emotions and my energy levels.

Our emotions and mental energy can be just as easily drained as our physical energy, and our bucket needs to be checked and replenished often throughout the day. By checking our emotional and physical energy daily, we can ensure that our bucket doesn't run empty when we're not looking and that we aren't tempted to buy instant credit to replace a temporary need. Examples of instant credit sources would include energy drinks and multiple coffee and sugary drinks, that give us a temporary boost before crashing and forcing us to buy more credit to keep us going. With all sources of instant credit, we end up paying back more in the end than we used in the first place. Using the energy we have and not overspending is a great way of monitoring our wellbeing.

In a similar way, you can continue going, not realising for example that being stressed out and depressed drains your emotional energy, impacting the energy you have for yourself and your child.

What Was the Point of It All?

I have written this book because I know firsthand the impact mental health issues have on us if they aren't managed in their earliest, mildest forms. Our bodies are always communicating; they're always speaking with us and telling us what they need. Often, especially in modern days, we don't listen. My family has a weakness for cancer and mental illness. Your family may have a weakness for diabetes or dementia. Each family has their own 'Achilles heel', a condition that will tell us when we need to change the way we live. It will tell us by manifesting as an illness or condition that we can overcome by stopping, listening to what is needed, and taking action to course-correct.

One of my young clients, 12-year-old Jimmy, used to lock himself in his room, only emerging to eat and drink. He regularly berated and blamed his parents for giving birth to him. Jim was a school refuser, and had been excluded when he was 11 from secondary school for being angry and throwing a chair at a teacher. Jimmy taunted and bullied his parents and smoked weed openly.

When Jimmy's parents approached me, they were desperate for help and support. Much of their furniture was broken, as Jimmy would get angry and take it out on the furniture or push the doors or walls. The father was, himself, on antidepressants. Jimmy's younger brother, who up until then had been the perfect child, had started misbehaving in class.
In our organisation, Julian Campbell Foundation (JCF) mentors are trained to support young people and their families. These mentors are people in the community who have relatives or friends that have suffered from mental

health difficulties and want to make a difference, supporting young people through difficult times in their life. In addition, another mentor along with a psychologist supports and advises each community mentor throughout the 12-week intervention to encourage the young person receiving support to move them closer to their goals much more quickly than if they were alone.

At JCF, we train mentors who go on to support children and their families. And so in this way, we provided support for Jimmy and his parents. Through working with our mentors, Jimmy learned to recognise his moods and take action. Within four weeks of refusing to leave the house, Jimmy went out for a walk with his mentor. Within eight weeks, Jimmy was back in education. By 12 weeks, the family had transformed. Jimmy started leaving the house with his family, and the relationships between him, his parents, and his brother had improved. Jimmy was able to identify and manage his moods and start looking at his future with hope instead of blaming his family.

So, in your life right now, what is your body telling you that you have been ignoring or hoping that it will go away? What is your child telling you that you haven't been listening to or thinking that it will soon pass? Listening to these messages and taking action will make the difference and transform situations in your life that you have been putting up with or tolerating. In our organization, these changes can take up to 12 weeks. However, with dedication and focus, you can transform your life in your own chosen time frame. Because new habits take two weeks to become fully incorporated into our way of being, it is my suggestion that you spend two weeks focusing on each chapter and applying the aspects you choose to your life.

CHAPTER 2
The BIG Solution Framework

'Our deepest fear is not that we are inadequate. Our deepest fear is that we are powerful beyond measure. It is our light, not our darkness, that most frightens us'.

Marianne Williamson

Here you are right now, with parts of your life that work and parts of your life that definitely do not, or at least do not work as well as you would like them to. You're ready to take on the latter and improve your life and the life of your child. You have an idea that you can overcome the difficulties you're having, if you had a little support and guidance to see you through to the other side. However, it is difficult to know exactly how to start and what you have to do to ensure that the ways your family deals with and manages the depression, anxiety, or schizophrenia don't get passed down to your children. You have depression, and although you have overcome it, you have concerns that your children may start learning dysfunctional ways of managing their moods and depression from you. For this, you decide, 'I'm going to make sure that my children get all the support and guidance they need to manage their wellbeing to make sure they don't fall prone to any of these illnesses later on in their life.'

Fifty percent of mental health difficulties in adulthood manifest before the age of 14 years old. If you start now, while your child is young, you have a chance of dealing with these difficulties before they can fully arise. The path toward happiness and wellbeing includes taking on new habits around developing emotional intelligence in your child, developing your own empathy, learning to forgive and finding self-love, the importance of keeping your word for you and your children, and modelling for them that you are what you eat as well as teaching them how to let go of disruptive behaviours.

So What's Next?

We will start our journey by learning how to be the change we wish to see. Empathy will help you look over to the other side of the fence and understand what your child is dealing with. By learning to manage your own emotions, you can help your child learn to monitor their moods and feelings and figure out how they can change their mood states with simple behaviours that they can use for a lifetime as well as pass on to their own children and future generations.

You will come to see that your child's behaviour is a mirror, a reflection of how you're being with them. Once you see your reflection clearly through the behaviour of others, including your children, it's easier to take action to improve your relationship with yourself and each and every person around you. You can get your power back.

'Talk is cheap': We will examine this phrase and explore whether we are belying what we say by exercising a lack of consistency and not following through on things we say we're going to do. It doesn't work to make a promise to yourself or a child and then renege on this promise based on changing emotions or moods. This not only undermines your authority, it also dishonours the very essence of who you are.

When we do what we say we will do, when we are consistent in our own lives and the lives of our children, we will see progress in every aspect of our lives: eating healthy foods, taking regular exercise, choosing actions that elevate mental wellbeing and emotional intelligence rather than those that dishonour our bodies or bring and/or exacerbate mental health difficulties. Consistency is key, as well as communicating and demonstrating what being consistent looks like to your children by setting clear boundaries and following through with the consequences of poor behaviour. Your child must understand that when you ask them to do something, you mean it, and that you have clear punishments (sanctions) when they refuse to do as you have asked.

In the following chapters, we'll walk through seven steps to get you and your family where you want to be. In each chapter, we'll look at our lives and evaluate them from the following perspectives:

- **Looking at the man in the mirror** – We start with looking at ourselves by using the others as a mirror to see our own previously hidden behaviours, which allows us the opportunity to change them. We learn to get in touch with our own moods and emotions and "be the change".
- **Whose fault is it anyway? It's not mine!** – This step shows us how to be accountable and take charge of our lives in a way that will empower us.

- **Where is the love?** – Where is our self-love? This chapter helps us find ourselves and fall in love with ourselves again on a whole new level.
- **It's not our fears, it's our power that we're afraid of** – If you have ever felt afraid, know that you can find your joy and power underneath it all. We'll look at ways of stepping into our power that leaves us and those around us with more freedom.
- **We are what we eat** – We'll explore the reasons why eating foods high in carbohydrates leaves us feeling tired and more prone to depression, and learn why changing our eating habits has a positive impact on our emotions and mood. Structuring and developing consistent mealtimes also helps strengthen family relationships.
- **Being consistent** - putting it all together and going from strength to strength, making time for yourself and your family in your daily schedule.
- **Key behaviours** – to avoid so you can continue to make progress and focus on development from strength to strength.

CHAPTER 3
What's the point of knowing how I feel?

'I'm looking at the man in the mirror'.
Michael Jackson

What is the point of knowing how you feel? It's important because when you know how you feel, you can then start searching for the reason you feel that way and that's how you find your solution.

In this chapter, we will look at your child's behaviour as a reflection of your own moods and emotions, and see how emotions show that there is a part of your past that isn't resolved.

Empathy, or Emotional intelligence

There are many things your child has to deal with while growing up, and it's easy to fall for the illusion that intelligence and education are the most important. They are certainly important to a degree. But there is another type of intelligence, emotional intelligence, that is even more important. Through emotional intelligence, children learn to foster better-quality relationships, are more focused in school, are better judges of character, and go on to have a greater range of career choices, working with and leading groups of people. Furthermore, children with highly developed emotional intelligence are more able to manage their behaviour and their mental wellbeing.

This is where you come in. Children are emotional sponges, and they absorb the atmosphere around them. Whether you mean to or not, you are modelling what your child will become. It's important to get in touch with yourself in order to determine whether what you are modelling is actually what you want your child to learn.

It begins with learning to recognise your own emotions and how to deal with them effectively. There's nothing wrong with feeling angry or upset, but it doesn't work to take action when angry. Do not try to suppress these emotions, either. When you acknowledge how you feel, these emotions will subside more quickly. When we blame ourselves and think something is wrong with us, we'll have a harder time listening to the answers that will guide us to the solution. Stop focusing on what is wrong and focus on what you need to change in yourself. Consider that your child is your reflection and your child, through their actions and behaviour, will always show you where you need to work on yourself to develop emotionally. Turn your focus onto yourself and your behaviour, identify and control your emotions, and improve your connection with your child.

How do I feel right now?

Why have you decided to follow this programme? What is your goal and your purpose? It could be any of these: 'I think my depression is affecting my son and I don't want him to have it', or 'I think my daughter could be depressed or anxious and this will help her', or 'I want to enjoy wellbeing and develop healthy habits to pass down to future generations of my family', or any other thoughts you may have. This purpose needs to be something that really inspires you and keeps you going when the going may get a little rough. Write it down so you can see it every day, in your diary, in the pages of a journal, or on your phone.

How is your life right now? Spend 10 minutes writing down a minimum of five things that describe your life right now, five things that you would like to change in your life and your relationship with your child. For example, you could decide, 'I want her to listen to me', 'I want us to stop fighting', or 'I wish I could like him'.

After writing your list, imagine that you have the relationship that you really want with your child. How would it be? Write down at least five sentences describing this. For example, 'I want us to be close', or 'I want him to really love me'. You can draw if this is a better way to illustrate your life. You may need time to think about this and collect your thoughts together, and if this is the case, you can come back to this tomorrow after you've had time to reflect.

Once you have your five sentences, keep them in a safe place where you can easily find them. When we work with clients, we generally recommend they repeat this exercise again in 12 weeks, so they can compare and see the progress that they've made, and I encourage you to do so, too.

How can my child get to understand how he feels?

There are tools that can help you identify your mood, and tools that you can use with your child. Can you imagine the advantages of identification of mood from a young age? Once children know how to identify what they are feeling, they're able to manage their moods, which develops their emotional intelligence. The mood meter, introduced by Jennings & Greenberg 2009 and developed at Yale University, has been used by teachers and young people alike throughout the school day to help them identify their moods. The mood meter below is a simplified version that uses colour to describe each mood with one word, and is more useful for younger children from ages 3-8. For example:

- The colour red section is associated with anger
- The colour blue section is associated with being sad
- The colour green section is associated with being calm
- The colour yellow section is associated with being happy

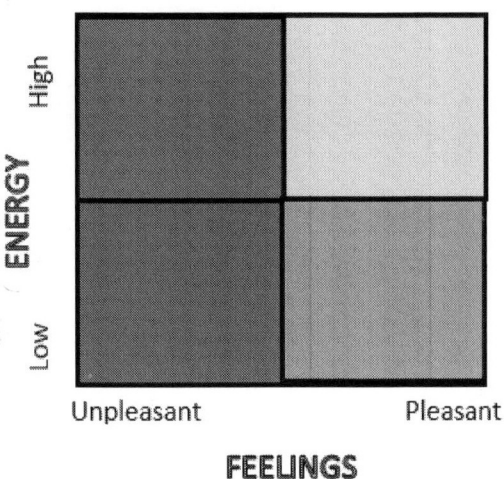

The mood meter uses a graph to measure how good we're feeling or our mood on the axis going across (the horizontal axis). We measure our energy level on the part of the graph going upwards (the vertical axis). Each thing that we measure, how good we're feeling and how much energy we have, can be measured from -5 (which would be a really low mood or low energy) to +5 (which would be a really great and positive mood or lots of energy).

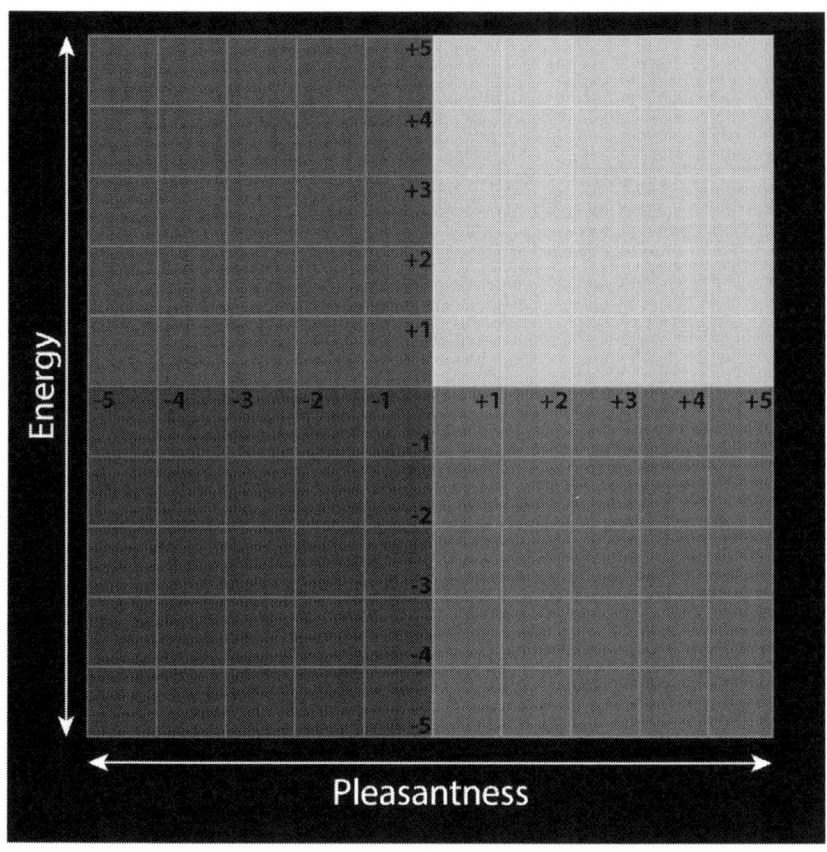

An example of a high energy mood for example, would be 'energised' (+3 on the graph). An example of a mood that is neither good nor bad, but neutral (0 pleasantness or 0 feelings). If we had around the same level of energy and were feeling really rubbish (a low mood), this would push us into the red section of the mood meter, making us 'worried' (-4 on the pleasantness axis going across). On the other hand, if we had the same amount of energy and we were feeling really positive, we would be in a 'pumped' mood (+3 on the pleasantness axis going across).

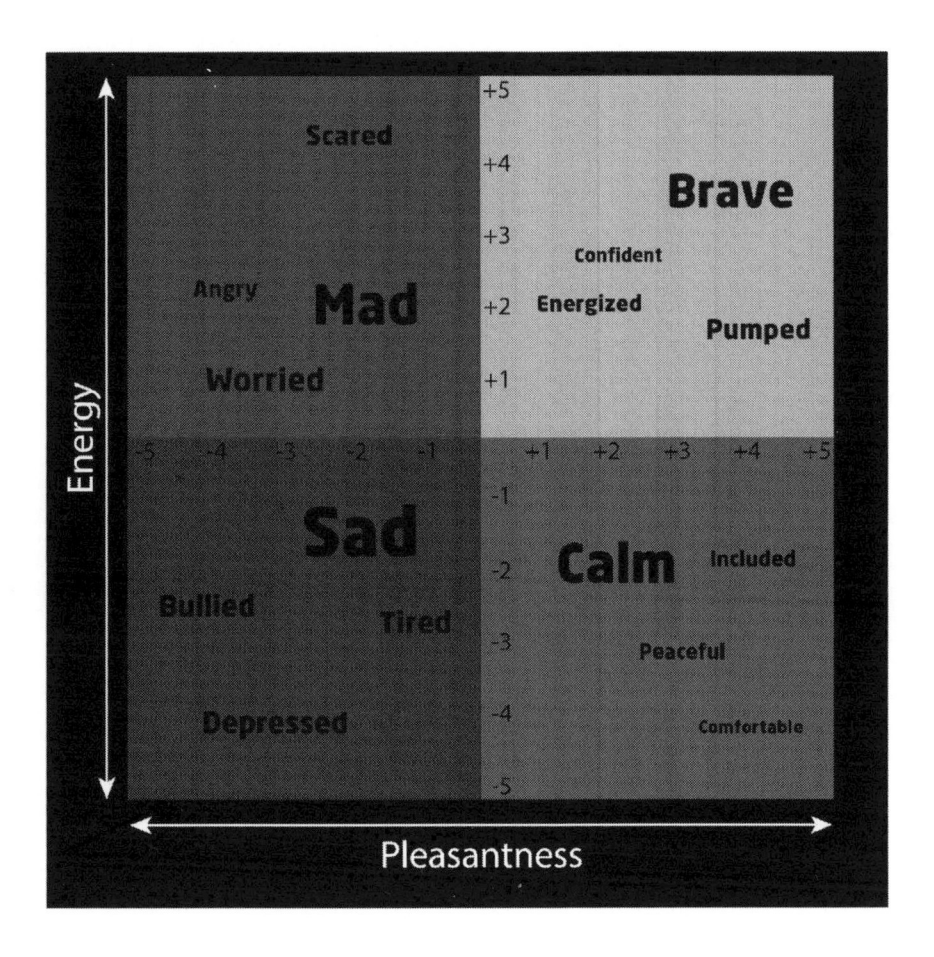

![Mood meter diagram showing a grid with Energy on the vertical axis and Pleasantness on the horizontal axis, divided into four quadrants: Mad (upper left) with Scared, Angry, Worried; Brave (upper right) with Confident, Energized, Pumped; Sad (lower left) with Bullied, Tired, Depressed; Calm (lower right) with Included, Peaceful, Comfortable.]

Look at the emotions of being 'worried' and 'pumped' for example. Both of them are around +3 on the horizontal axis and are high-energy emotions, however, the 'pumped' emotion has a higher degree of pleasantness with +3 and the 'worried' emotion has a lower degree of pleasantness or negative emotion of -3.

What do you do once you've identified each emotion? Jennings & Greenberg developed five RULER skills to help us identify and understand our emotions. RULER is an acronym to help children Recognise, Understand, Label, Express, and Regulate their emotions:

> **R**ecognise: How are you feeling? How do you know you are feeling that way? Can you show me a _____ face?
>
> **U**nderstand: What happened that led you to feel this way? What happens that makes you feel _____?
>
> **L**abel: What word best describes how you are feeling? Where would you put this on the mood meter? What is the name of this feeling?
>
> **E**xpress: How can you express what you are feeling for this time and place? What else can you do when you are feeling _____?
>
> **R**egulate: What can you do to maintain your feeling (if you want to continue feeling this way), or shift your feeling (if you do not want to continue feeling this way)? What could you do to help a friend who is feeling _____? When you feel _____, what do you do?

These steps can help you start a dialogue to identify and change your mood and your child's mood.

Here's what this looks like in action: Charlotte, a 38-year-old mother, uses the mood meter daily with her 8-year-old son Dillan. Each morning and at intervals throughout the day, Charlotte assesses her emotions and thinks about how her feelings will affect her relationship with her son. One morning, she measures her emotion on the mood meter as being 'anxious' (that is energy +4 and pleasantness -4).

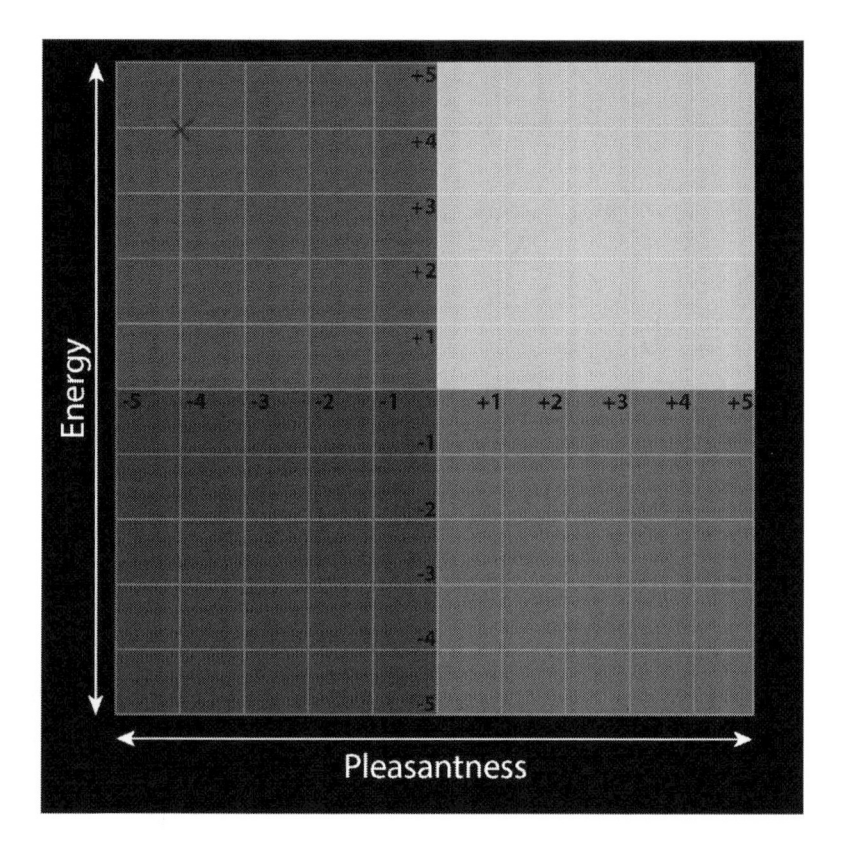

She tells Dillan that she is feeling a little anxious today and explains why; that she's expecting some important results from her doctor, who she's visiting today. The advantages of this are that Charlotte is showing Dillan how to be more empathic, and she's also building his emotional intelligence. By sharing how she's feeling with Dillan, Charlotte is moving along the positive scale of pleasantness/feelings. In addition, Charlotte walks to school with Dillan and walks through the park to reduce the energy she has that's making her feel anxious thus, reducing her anxiety.

Charlotte's graph will show that she has reduced her stress after her walk and speaking about what she's dealing with, changing her mood intensity to feeling uneasy instead of frightened. (The before and after graphs show Charlotte's change in mood).

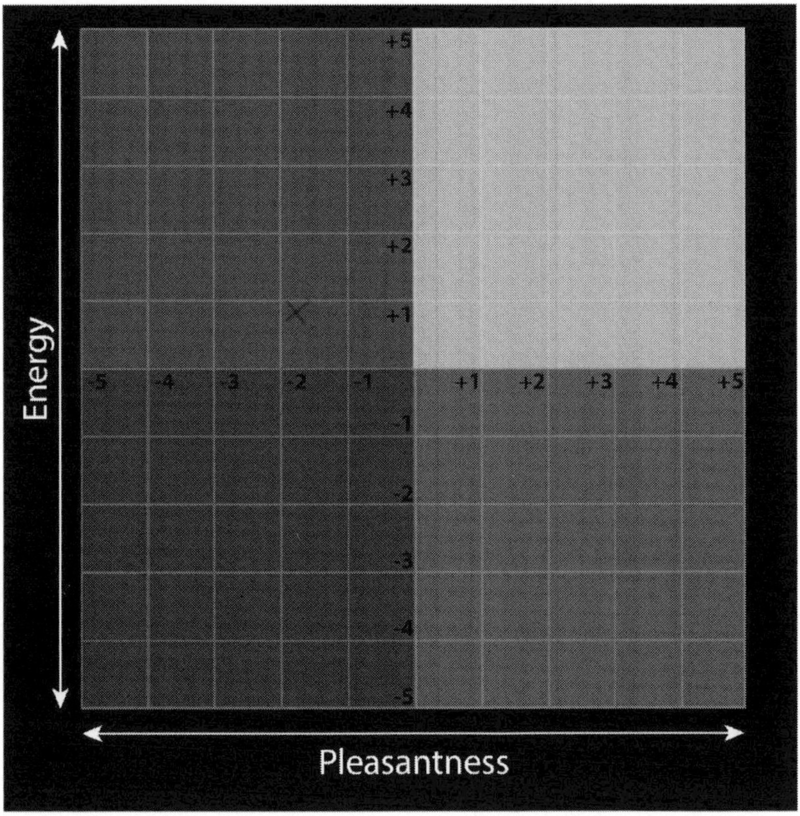
Energy
Pleasantness
+5
+4
+3
+2
+1
-5
-4
-3
-2
-1
+1
+2
+3
+4
+5
-1
-2
-3
-4
-5

Start using the mood meter and recording your mood every morning, afternoon, and evening. Also, use the mood meter (see below as a guide) with your child at least three times a day for the next two weeks, using each of the five RULER skills steps.

Mood Meter

Y-axis: Energy
X-axis: Pleasantness

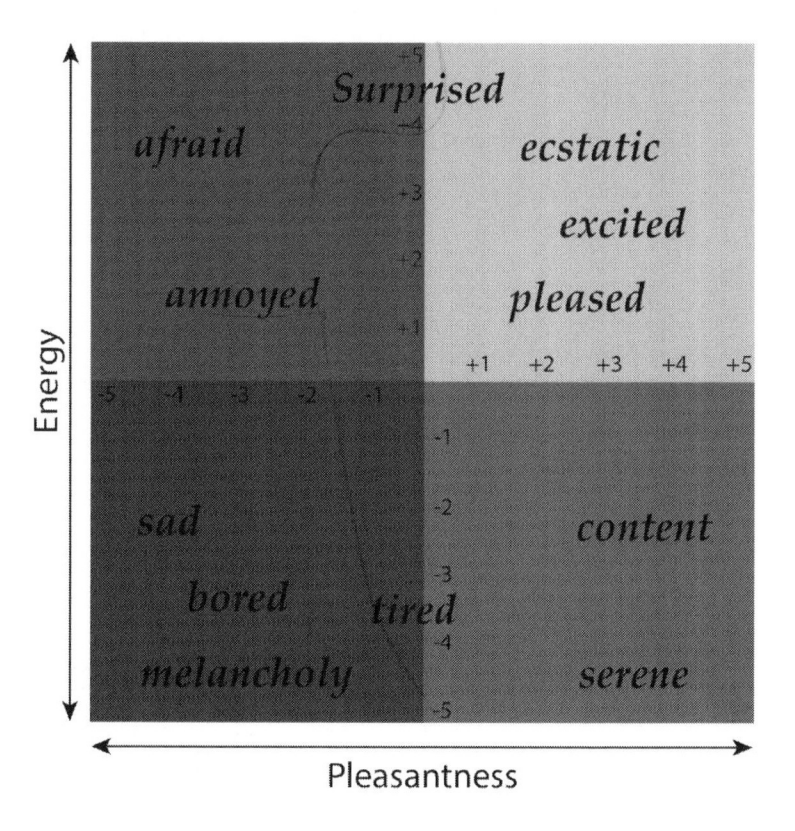

Upper-left quadrant (high energy, unpleasant): afraid, annoyed, Surprised
Upper-right quadrant (high energy, pleasant): ecstatic, excited, pleased
Lower-left quadrant (low energy, unpleasant): sad, bored, melancholy, tired
Lower-right quadrant (low energy, pleasant): content, serene

How do you start using the mood meter? You could download the app on www.moodmeterapp.com, or design and make your own mood meter chart if you're feeling creative. Alternatively, you could get a whiteboard from the pound shop, put it on the wall in your kitchen, and start plotting. From October 2018, you can download and use the JCF MoodApp from our website, www.juliancampbellfoundation.org. The two mood meter graphs here (above and below) give you some examples of feelings to help develop your descriptions.

				M	Surprised	Upbeat	Motivated	Ecstatic
				O	Hyper	Cheerful	Inspired	Elated
				O	Energized	Lively	Optimistic	Thrilled
				D	Pleasant	Joyful	Proud	Blissful
M	**O**	**O**	**D**	**M**	**E**	**T**	**E**	**R**
Disgusted	Disappointed	Glum	Ashamed	**E**	Blessed	At Ease	Content	Fulfilled
Mortified	Alienated	Mopey	Apathetic	**T**	Humble	Secure	Chill	Grateful
Embarrassed	Excluded	Timid	Drained	**E**	Calm	Satisfied	Relaxed	Carefree
Alone	Down	Bored	Tired	**R**	Relieved	Restful	Tranquil	Serene

Put your measurements into a little notebook or something small that you can carry around with you and make notes of any changes to reflect on later. Record any changes in your journal. If you're using an app, you can record everything without paper.

What have you seen for yourself in the last two weeks?

What do you do to shift your mood when you feel a negative mood? For example, do you speak to a friend, listen to your favourite music, write a poem, take 10 minutes to yourself? Spend time on an activity, leisure activity, or pastime that you love? Write any more interventions you put in place here.

What do you do to change your energy when you have low energy? Drink more water? Go for a walk around the block or the park? Take a handful of cashews or almonds (for a boost of protein and magnesium)? Have a nap or have an early night? Listen to your favourite tune?

What have you seen for your child?

What do you do with your child when s/he's in a negative mood or low energy? Do you speak with them to find out where they're at on mood meter and what they're dealing with? Are they doing any activities such as dance, classes, or groups, learning an instrument, or something that is fostering their self-expression?

Can you see any connection between your moods and theirs? You may have noticed that your child reflects your mood. Furthermore, when you take steps to change your mood, then this, too, has an impact on your child.

Your child is very much your mirror and an external measure of your own moods and emotions.

Well done for taking the first step in building empathy in yourself and your child. In the next chapter, we will look at how we can develop our skills of empathy by looking at a crucial ingredient, being responsible, and how this will further empower us.

CHAPTER 4
Rules for peace and harmony

'There is nothing enlightened about shrinking so that other people won't feel insecure around you. We are all meant to shine, as children do.'

Marianne Williamson

In Chapter 3, we looked at your own moods and the moods of your child. You will have found that while you are two different beings, your moods are likely very similar. Your child is your reflection and is showing you your own emotions. What does this mean? This means that essentially, you are responsible.

When I say responsible, I mean that it starts with you, that your family's mood derives from you as its source. We have a natural tendency to blame another for certain situations; this is our default mechanism working, and this is a normal way of thinking. Blaming someone else for something that happens in our life is a way of giving away our power and remaining a victim. When we're a victim, we feel powerless and unable to overcome the situation that we're in.

By taking responsibility, we can see how we have contributed to every situation. I'm not saying that whether you're a victim or not is the truth. There are many truths out there. However, looking at things through the filter of being responsible is a truth will help you take positive and bold steps in this area (and other areas) of your life to give you power and peace. The great thing here is that all you need to do is work on yourself and your child will follow suit. It all begins with you.

In this chapter, we'll look at how all the negative emotions that you are feeling get in the way of the love you have for yourself, and that the behaviour you see in your child that you don't like is actually something about you that you don't like and you can't see it in yourself. The good news here is that when we see it in our child, we can act on that emotion, overcome it, and feel more peaceful, falling in love with ourselves and our child on a whole new level.

Cem, nine years old, was terrorising his family when his father contacted us. The father had been working full-time, but due to a work accident had lost his job. The family was struggling financially, and Cem's father was taking medication due to a diagnosis of clinical depression. Cem spent the majority of his time in his room and wasn't engaging with anyone. When the family went out together, for shopping, or to do things as a family, Cem refused to go. Cem's smaller brother was well-behaved and did not cause any problems.

Cem's parents told us that he taunted them in their home. When his mother was in the kitchen, sometimes Cem would enter and pour spices or flour or salt into the dinner as she was cooking. One time, Cem told his father that if he smoked marijuana, it would be better than the tablets his dad was taking. He would regularly blame his mother for giving birth to him. However, at school Cem was well-behaved, and so the parents didn't know who to speak with about their situation. Their difficulty was compounded by the fact that the parents did not speak English and couldn't communicate their needs. They found our advert in a local Turkish newspaper.

Specially trained mentors in our organisation started supporting this family, along with providing a mentor for Cem over the next 12 weeks. Our mentors discovered that Cem's family existed in a climate of fear, not wanting to rock the boat for fear that one of Cem's violent outbursts would lead to more broken doors and furniture.

Cem's parents were frightened, a negative mood and low energy on the mood meter. Through our weekly sessions, they were invited to examine their feelings and talk about how they could improve their mood and increase their energy. It helped them greatly to speak with us; in turn, we provided them with the support they needed to set up a framework for Cem to follow, a framework of discipline in which there were clear and strict boundaries and consistent consequences for going beyond them. We also taught Cem's parents to communicate in low, calm voices.

Over time, the climate of fear became an atmosphere of hope. Cem responded well to his mentor, and they soon started leaving the house and going for walks, something that Cem hadn't done for the last year. With regular support, Cem's parents got out of the negative mood/negative energy rut and were more peaceful and content. However, this is an example of where the parent's emotions and what they're dealing with can impact the child. Cem did everything he did for attention, and although it was negative attention, it was attention nonetheless. Through being bold, positive, and hopeful, Cem's parents were able to transform their situation and overcome the hardships that they were suffering.

This underscores why, now that you have started speaking with your child about their moods on a regular basis and can help them understand what it is that they need to do to shift their mood, it's essential to look for the deeper need when your child is quiet, grumpy, hyperactive, or just generally out of sync. There's usually a reason for this.

Being naughty is a good attention-grabber as well as a great way of triggering us as parents into action. Our young can be master manipulators and trigger us into reacting by shouting and blaming, which promotes overwhelm, decreases power, and increases anxiety. I say master manipulators because children can tap into any area or emotion that shows you have something unresolved. What is it that is unresolved for you? Whatever it is, your child will find it and manipulate you over this.

Cem, for example, bullied his parents and blamed them for his birth. He told them that he wished he had never been born. This is an extremely difficult situation and of course, something difficult to respond to. However, in this case, Cem was crying for his parent's attention, but because he was triggering their fear, they didn't know where to start. When they worked together to start giving him positive attention, showing him their love instead of fear, and being consistent with their punishments, they overcame this difficult time. If they felt themselves becoming triggered, they waited until they were in a positive mood and informed Cem that they would discipline him later on.

In the next section, we will look at putting rules in place to increase your power and bring peace and harmony to your life.

Whose fault is it if it's not mine?

When I started working as a science teacher, it was a real struggle. The way my classes behaved were not how I imagined them going in my head. I took many things for granted. Although I planned every minute of my lesson, what I would be doing and what the students would be doing, there were still moments of disruption in my class. I had to constantly evaluate my classes and think, 'It would be even better if I did…'. I continued to do this until I found methods that worked for me in all areas of my teaching. It took me about three years to develop my teaching skills so that my classes behaved exactly how I wanted them to behave. I used assertive discipline', which meant rewarding good behaviour and not focusing on poor behaviour. This procedure involved making a note of students who didn't follow one of the five main rules of my classroom and openly praising and rewarding the ones who did. My rules were:

1. Attend all your classes on time
2. Follow instructions the first time given
3. Raise your hand if you need to speak and don't shout
4. Complete your homework on time
5. Keep your hands, feet, and objects to yourself

My classes transformed into peace and tranquility. I was surprised, but happy that I could then teach what I wanted to. We played many games, had fun, and most importantly, the students enjoyed my lessons and went on to achieve very good grades. When I started out I was, in my opinion, a weak teacher because things were not as I wanted them to be. However, after great reviews from OFSTED, Office for Standards in Education, Children's Services, and Skills, I went into consultancy and I was advised that other teachers should see my teaching to learn from me. The transformations in my teaching and in my classrooms were achieved by my looking each time at my performance to see what I could improve.

In a similar way, I want you to choose five rules that would transform your household. I suggest you choose just five, as too many rules could get confusing. You know what they are and also, it really does depend on what you want to achieve in your home. For example, you could choose the following rules:

1. Do what mum and dad say first time
2. Tell the truth
3. Ask permission before you go anywhere
4. Put things away that you take out
5. Keep your hands, feet, objects, and anger to yourself

You can find more examples of these kinds of rules on www.babycentre.co.uk.

Once you have found the five that work for you – and you will know what they are, because they'll be calling out to you – share them with your children. Explain the reason for each one, For example, doing what mum and dad say the first time is important because if you start shouting, this means that you haven't listened to their parents' instructions the first time and are turning it into an argument. It is important to let your child know that although you have listened to what they have said and you acknowledge it, you nonetheless want them to do what you ask the first time with no arguments. Be bold and follow these guidelines for at least the two weeks it will take to instill new changes and turn them into new habits. It will be difficult at first, because any new rule takes time. Children are going to push the boundaries – this is what we all do, adults and children alike. Stay consistent and do not change your mind, as this will convey the message that your rules are not workable and that your child can push the boundaries and get away with things. It is also important to develop your children's emotional intelligence; as they grow and get used to a system that has rules and defined consequences for breaking them, it won't work for them in the long run if they feel they can disregard them and get away with it. Each rule has a sanction. Stick to it.

During this time, continue to map your and your child's moods in your journal or on the fridge in your kitchen or communal area, making time to speak with them to find out what they're dealing with, where they are on the mood meter, and how to change their mood. By now, you are illustrating your moods and emotions by speaking with your child, telling them how you feel, and why. Continue to model the change you wish to see in your child.

One of our mentors and I were supporting a teenager and her family in enforcing rules and upholding sanctions. Samantha, 15, had been excluded from school for being violent. When we started supporting her, Samantha wasn't in school and refused to attend any centres for education to complete her studies. Samantha was staying in her room through the day and terrorising her family, refusing to follow any rules that her parents made. If she stayed in the house, she would regularly stay up through the night watching films. She isolated herself, making friends on line and going out to meet them without her parents' knowledge. This continued despite her parents request not to do this. Her parents were really concerned for Samantha's safety, and didn't know what do to help her. This had a negative impact on the entire household with arguments between Samantha and her parents, ending up in her leaving their house and disappearing overnight.

We started supporting Samantha and her family. We suggested that the next time Samantha got angry and started verbally abusing her family and threatening them physically, that her family tell Samantha to stop. If she continued, we recommended that they call the police and report Samantha's behaviour as disturbing the peace of the family, household, and their surroundings. Samantha stopped the verbal abuse and left the house, coming back later in silence. This happened one more time. The final time, three weeks later, Samantha continued her behaviour as she had before and started getting violent, along with cursing. I was with the parents (who were beside themselves with all of this) as I (on their behalf) made the decision to contact the police and the hospital to help us manage the situation.

They turned up several hours later. By this time, Samantha was in her room. The police questioned Samantha and took her to hospital. Samantha was only there for a few hours; she arrived around 9.00 pm and was discharged at 4.00 the following morning. When Samantha returned, she was a different person. We continued to mentor and support her, and her family and Samantha didn't repeat that behaviour again. Her parents had warned her what they would do if she continued threatening them, and they followed it through. Because of this, the atmosphere in the household lifted as things transformed and the parents took back their power.
In the next chapter, we'll look at how we can optimise peace and tranquility in our relationships by putting simple structures in place.

CHAPTER 5 - Self-care

'Tell me what you eat and I will tell you what you are'.

Anthelme Brillat-Savarin

Are We Active Enough?

In the first half of the book, we looked at our own behaviours and environment to see how we can change it. We can only change the parts of our environment that we have control over, we cannot change other people. As we're accountable for each thought that we have and each mood, stopping these negative thoughts and replacing them with positive ones will transform the world around us. The more responsibility we can take for our relationships, the more we can look at the impact of our behaviour without blaming ourselves. Seeing our child's behaviour as a reflection of ourselves gives us back our power to create lasting change.

We can take many actions around our health to ensure we improve our own mood and concentration as well as that of our child. Everyone needs to take care of their wellbeing, especially to ensure that our emotional health and mental health are robust. All families have some disposition towards one type of illness or another, such as heart attacks, diabetes, or cancer for example. As I've said, my family has a tendency towards mental health difficulties, which means that we must be aware of our health, fitness, and what we're putting into our bodies.

Have you noticed that people who have mental health difficulties as a rule are also extremely intelligent? The fact that we have these illnesses in the gene pool must mean that the people who have them (and their genes) are very attractive! Family members who have a tendency to have mental health difficulties (anxiety, stress, depression, schizophrenia, bipolar, ADHD, etc.) and are intelligent must take care of their brains. In this and the next chapter, we will be looking at the importance of eating the correct foods as well as the best type of exercise to promote our wellbeing.

The UK guidelines recommend that a child take one hour of movement each day, but at this moment, only 9 percent of our kids are getting their recommended amount of exercise. What is more common is that children are spending four to seven minutes a day moving around, and seven hours in front of a screen.
Studies have shown that children who play outside are happier, more attentive, and less anxious than children who stay inside more. Also, children who engage in moderate to vigorous physical activity between the ages of six and eight have fewer symptoms of depression two years later. Moderate exercise includes cycling, gardening, dancing, jogging, playing tennis, swimming, low-impact aerobics, and walking. Exercise has been shown to decrease muscle tension, release feel-good chemicals, improve brain functioning, combat behaviour disorders, and boost emotional wellbeing due to the endorphins that are released during exercise. Endorphins are chemicals, or neurotransmitters, that send electrical signals around the nervous system. They're made in the brain, and their job is to fight pain and fight stress. A very useful chemical to have an abundance of in our bodies, I think!

How much exercise is your child taking right now? If your child is spending four to seven minutes a day moving around, then you can increase their activity week by week by five to ten minutes. As adults, we are recommended to walk for 40 minutes each day. This doesn't have to be all at once, you can take a ten-minute walk four times a day if you wish. You can spend time playing with the kids and become physically active as a family, taking hikes, cycling, walking, or skating. Let your child cycle to school, and allow them to have active time after school.

Which activities does your child like doing? Swimming, football, basketball, dancing, gymnastics, or others? Or creative outlets such as writing, playing a musical instrument, or dancing? Attending classes together can develop new skills and be lots of fun, as well as improve the relationship you have with your children.

How many minutes a day do you and your children take moderate activity? Do you already walk to school in the morning, or is that something that you could start doing now? This week, continue to record your and your child's mood four times a day. What do you notice? Are there any changes in your mood? Also, what about the mood of your child?

In Chapter 5, I spoke about a young boy, Cem, who refused to leave the house for one year. He went to school sometimes, but as he found it difficult to leave the house, he stayed more and more in his room. Within 12 weeks of providing Cem support, he was attending school full-time and going on small outdoor excursions, at first only with his mentor and then, gradually on his own and with family. In addition, Cem started to play football again and so was exercising for recommended one hour a day. His moods transformed and his depression lifted. Now, Cem continues to be more sociable and is attending college, training to be an engineer as he had always wanted.

Making sure you're moving around each day is crucial as within two weeks, the effects of this activity can be compared to taking an antidepressant.

Feeding Our Brains the Right Food

We have looked at the importance of maintaining our brain in tiptop condition, which is crucial to promoting our wellbeing. When we have been gifted a brain that is more active than the average brain, we really need to spend time and effort giving it the best treatment and fuel possible. There's much research on the genetic link between intelligence and mental disorder and also links to suggest that depression decreases intelligence. Whatever the story, we must feed our brains with the correct food for it to provide us and our loved ones with the mindset we need to live well and have the lives we dream of.

Today's Western diet is full of processed foods that are doing damage to our children and their physical and mental health. I've seen our kids at dinner time buying McDonald's, fish and chips, and other processed foods that don't have any nutritional value and damage wellbeing. I'm not saying that they should never do this, it's just important to balance these foods and not eat them all of the time. Both our wellbeing and mental illness are influenced by diet. When comparing the Western diet with that of the Japanese diet, studies show that the Japanese way of eating prevents depression by up to 35 percent due to their diet of unprocessed food, fermented foods, and natural probiotics. We will talk about the importance of probiotics in this chapter. So what foods are better for our brains and why do we need them?

What Can We Eat to Make a Difference Now?

Vitamin B

Vitamin B's play an important role in manufacturing brain chemicals that affect our mood, assisting in nerve growth and development, improving communication between nerve cells, and providing emotional and mental energy. Low levels of B12 and B6 and folate (vitamin 9) have been linked to anxiety and depression.

Vitamin D

Vitamin D, or the 'sunshine vitamin', plays an important role in bone health and has recently been found important for other areas of health, also. Vitamin D is found on the surface of cells instructing them to act in a certain way, for example, to die or divide. Vitamin D can be absorbed through the skin and, depending on your skin tone, you need more exposure to the sun to get your quota. Ten minutes is enough for fair complexions, with up to a one-hour exposure for darker skins. Absorption of vitamin D assists with the absorption of calcium, helping to build strong bones, teeth, and muscles. Several studies have suggested that Seasonal Affective Disorder (SAD) may be due to the changing levels of vitamin D, which impact the serotonin levels in the brain.

While I think that your 40- to 60-minute daily walk will generate enough vitamin D for you and your child, respectively, these foods can also help boost your vitamin D: fish like salmon, sardines, mackerel, and tuna; raw milk: caviar; eggs; and mushrooms.

Omega-3 oils

Omega-3 oils build brain cell membranes and reduce brain inflammation, both important to make new brain cells, improve mood and memory, and protect us against brain disorders such as dementia and depression as well as reducing the symptoms of ADHD in children. Omega-3s improve focus and the ability to finish tasks, and they decrease hyperactivity, impulsiveness, restlessness, and aggression. Low omega-3 levels have been reported in people with mental disorders, but supplements can reduce the frequency of mood swings and relapses in people with schizophrenia and bipolar as well as decreasing violent behaviour. The following foods have sources of zinc:

- Salmon
- Flaxseed oil (cold-pressed)
- Walnuts and walnut oil
- Fish roe
- Mackerel (oily fish)
- Oysters
- Soybeans
- Spinach
- Egg yolks
- Halibut, herring, trout
- Tuna

Which foods do you eat already? If you already eat four of these eight, then that's a great start. It would be great to eat fish twice a week, which can be cooked pretty quickly with minimum preparation.

Zinc

Zinc is an essential mineral that is found in our brain in higher quantities than elsewhere in the body. Deficiencies of zinc can lead to symptoms of depression, ADHD, difficulties with learning and memory, aggression, seizure, and violence. Zinc cannot be stored in the body for long periods of time, so it's important to eat zinc on a regular basis. The following foods have sources of zinc:

- Lamb
- Pumpkin seeds
- Grass-fed beef
- Chickpeas
- Cocoa powder
- Cashews
- Mushrooms
- Spinach
- Chicken

Which foods do you eat already? If there are already four of these eight foods in your diet, then that's a great start.

Calcium

Calcium deficiency is strongly linked to depression. It is already well known that calcium is really important for strong teeth and bones and that also our heart, muscles and nerves need calcium to function. However, calcium as also important for regulating mood, and has sedative and calming effects. Calcium needs to be consumed with fat in order to be used in the body. So for example, normal full-fat milk is a good source of calcium, but the calcium in skimmed milk is a waste, as the calcium will not be absorbed. The following foods have sources of calcium:

- Almonds
- Brazil nuts

- Dairy products like milk, yoghurt, and cheese
- Sardines
- Flax seeds
- Dark leafy greens such as spinach, kale, turnips, collard greens
- Green snap beans, broccoli, cooked okra, Chinese cabbage

Which foods do you eat already? If there's already four of these eight in your diet, then that's a great start.

Here are some other foods that really make a difference:

- Eggs are great because they have omega-3 oils and zinc to keep us alert and energised in order to regulate our metabolism and sugar level
- Avocado has the B vitamin folate, which is great to fight depression, tryptophan to boost our mood, and Vitamin B6 to relieve stress
- Sweet potatoes have the B Vitamin folate to fight depression
- Folate acid, Vitamin B 12 is important for pregnant women and all of us as it is important in making new cells, hair, skin, nails, and in supporting the liver and red blood production. Folate is found in leafy green vegetables, spinach and kale.
- Yoghurt with calcium to ease mood swings and eases depression and anxiety.
- Nuts such as walnuts and almonds, flax seed, olive oil, fresh basil, oily fish, salmon, trout, mackerel, anchovies, and sardines have omega-3 fatty acids, which decrease the inflammation that can cause arthritis, asthma, heart conditions, and certain types of cancer.

What is the link between the stomach and the brain?

The latest research is showing that the stomach and brain are much closely linked than previously thought. Our state of mind is connected to our gut because our gut uses the same chemicals as the brain and communicates with it. Our brain works hard day and night without rest, and needs optimum fuel to help us with our moods.

The best fuel that impacts our mood is the neurochemical transmitter (fuel) serotonin. Serotonin helps us sleep, inhibits pain, and regulates our appetite and moods by limiting inflammation. But how can it be that 95 percent of serotonin is produced in the gut if it fuels the brain? Our gut can be called the 'second brain', as it influences our mood and our wellbeing, and the microbes, the 'good bacteria' in our gut, play an important role in making serotonin. Therefore, we need to take good care of our microbes and make sure that we have lots of them at all times!
So how can we do this? What is good bacteria and what is the difference between 'good' and 'bad' bacteria? Another name for good bacteria is probiotics. Probiotics have a beneficial impact on our bodies because they prevent the bad bacteria from entering our body through the lining our intestines. In addition, they break down foods so we can use them in our bodies, produce several nutrients including vitamin K and B6, B12, niacin, and folic acid, and help us absorb calcium and magnesium. Therefore, we need to ensure that these nutrients are absorbed into our bodies, building strong bones and muscles. Bad bacteria, on the other hand, can cause upset stomach, bloating, swelling, and wind. In addition, the bad bacteria produces chemicals that damage the intestinal lining, resulting in 'leaky gut', which allows bacteria and other undesirables to get into our bloodstream and impact our moods and the way we physically feel. Studies have also

shown that an excess of bad bacteria can make us fat. Obese and diabetic patients have fewer good bacteria in their gut.

If we're not careful what we eat, we inadvertently kill off the good bacteria and feed the bad bacteria, causing a misbalance in our gut that impacts our moods. The trick is increasing the good bacteria and decrease the bad, which we do in three ways:

- Cutting down on eating foods that may be harming us
- Eating more of the foods that increase the good bacteria in our gut
- Taking a supplement to do the same as eating the right foods to increase the good bacteria

Cutting down on eating foods that may be harming us

Cutting down on eating certain foods that may be harming us is definitely a good start, as these foods increase the bad bacteria and destroy the good bacteria. What are the foods that are harmful?

- crisps
- ready-made meals
- chocolate
- refined sugar
- high-fat dairy
- cakes
- biscuits
- sweets
- ice cream

These have refined sugars and are harmful to our brain, impairing its functioning and worsening mood disorders. Which foods do you eat already? If there are already four or more of these eight in your diet, then you need to reduce them week by week. Eating an occasional treat, maybe once a week, is ok, but too much really does have a negative impact on the wellbeing of you and your child.

Eating more of the foods that increase the good bacteria in our gut

What are the foods that we need to be eating to increase that optimum fuel in our brains? Some sources of good bacteria are:

- asparagus
- garlic
- onions
- firm bananas
- legumes such as chickpeas, lentils, and kidney beans
- vinegars
- probiotic foods such as Yakult
- fermented foods such as sauerkraut, pickles, kimchi
- probiotic supplements

Taking a supplement to increase the good bacteria

Taking a supplement can do the same as eating the right foods to increase the good bacteria, and while there are many places you can buy them, I do advocate gaining levels of good bacteria through healthy eating, as you are modelling the behaviour you wish your child to adopt.

Which foods do you eat already? If there are already four of these eight, then that's a great start. Perhaps you already cook regularly using garlic and onions, or cook vegetables to eat with other foods. If so, good job. If not, choose a minimum of three of these foods that you can include in your diet this week. I'd say a probiotic drink and bananas would be a great start, as children love them!

Putting it all together

So putting all of this together, how often do you eat as a family? Once a day or more, or once a week or more? There are many researched benefits of eating as a family, including increased communication and wellbeing, modelling table manners, expanding your child's knowledge of foods, consuming more nourishing meals, becoming self-sufficient, preventing destructive behaviours, improved grades, and financial savings.

Communication and wellbeing

Mealtimes promote conversations about the day, learning from each other, and giving your children extra attention, warmth, security, and love, as well as a feeling of belonging. The experience of eating together can be a unifying experience for all of the family.

Modelling table manners

Family mealtimes are the perfect time to model table manners, meal etiquette, and social skills. Keep the mood light, relaxed, and loving, and try not to overtly instruct, or be critical.

Expanding your child's knowledge of foods

Expand your child's knowledge of foods by encouraging them to eat without forcing, coercing, or bribing. It's best to introduce a new food alongside some of the favourites. Remember that it can take eight to ten exposures to a new food before it is accepted, so be patient. Trying a new food is like starting a new hobby. It expands our child's knowledge, experience, and skill. Here is your opportunity to try new dishes using the ingredients we have spoken about in this chapter, ingredients that will promote wellbeing. Your child can choose a new recipe from a cookbook, website, or magazine.

Nourishing meals

Meals prepared and eaten at home are usually more nutritious, as they contain more fruits, vegetables, and dairy products with additional nutrients such as fiber, calcium, vitamins A and C, and folate. Home-cooked meals are not usually fried or highly salted, plus fizzy and sweet drinks consumption are usually lower at the dinner table.

Becoming self-sufficient

Becoming self-sufficient is a great advantage, as many children are missing out on the importance of knowing how to plan and prepare meals. Understanding basic cooking, baking, and food preparation is a necessity for being self-sufficient. Involve your family in menu planning, grocery shopping, and food preparation. If your child is attending nursery, they can tear lettuce and set the table. Older children can pour milk, peel vegetables, and mix batter. Teenagers can dice, chip, bake, and grill. Working as a team puts the meal on the table faster, as well as making everyone more responsible and accepting of the outcome. Improved eating habits come with 'ownership' of a meal.

Prevents destructive behaviours

Research shows that frequent family dinners (five or more a week) are associated with lower rates of smoking, drinking, and illegal drug use in pre-teens and teenagers, compared to families that eat together two or fewer times per week. Even as older children's schedules get more complicated, it is important to make an effort to eat more together. Scheduling (as spoken about earlier in this book) is a must.

Improved grades

Children do better in school when they eat more meals with their parents and family. Teenagers who eat dinner four or more times per week with their families have higher academic performance compared with teenagers who eat with their families two or fewer times per week.

Saving money

Meals purchased away from home cost two to four times more than prepared at home.

Today, it is common that due to scheduling, commitments, and activities, families eat out several times each week. However, eating breakfast together is a great way to start the day, to speak about how you feel, and gauge how your child feels on the mood meter. Also, eating together (without the television if possible) is a great way to evaluate how the day has gone, especially after school, and can really punctuate the end of the day. You may not be able to do this every day, as you may have constraints with work. Also, allowing your child to contribute to making the meal in some way will contribute to the enjoyment of the meal. If this is the case, make an effort to eat together as often as possible. By preparing meals together, your child is also taking responsibility and will be more likely to cook for themselves when they're independent. This is just as well, as the nutritional content is much, much higher.

Sharing dinner together can give a sense of identity, ease day-to-day conflicts, and establish traditions, memories, and behaviours that can last a lifetime.

We have seen in this chapter the foods that promote mental health and wellbeing. As I said at the beginning of this chapter, the Western diet is known for its richness in over-processed foods. The impact of a poor diet is well-documented, and increases the risk of cancer, diabetes, and heart conditions. It is crucial to know these same foods have a detrimental impact on our moods and mental health, with mounting evidence to support this every day. We're living in a fast society, and raising our children in these conditions, it is important that we set them up to survive and flourish. Cooking together using the foods discussed in this chapter would be a great thing to do as you're also bonding emotionally and spend quality time with your child. Putting in place even one or two of these tips will make a big difference in your lives and set your child up for the rest of his or her life.

CHAPTER 6
What are your key actions to avoid or drop?

'The truth of the matter is that you always know the right thing to do. The hard part is doing it'.

Robert Schuller

What can I drop now to make a difference?

This chapter will outline a few of the major players here, things that we do that don't really help with our wellbeing, have a negative impact on our relationship with our child, and are modelling behaviours we don't want our child to adopt.

Taking drugs and alcohol

Life is fast, and many of us have had things happen to us in the past that have been really difficult to get over. Sometimes we turn to our friends for comfort, but this isn't always enough for us to overcome what we're dealing with. It's commonplace in our society to find ways of taking away the pain. This may include using substances like heroin, marijuana, alcohol, or prescription drugs to help us through.

After being a victim of physical assault, I struggled with accepting it and made it mean all kinds of things about me. Smoking marijuana became a way of numbing the pain and escaping from my own thoughts. It took stopping drugs to come to the realisation that it was something that happened way back in my past and it was not happening now, so I didn't need to continue anymore.

I know it's a difficult situation and it is a tough one, because when we do this, we're modelling to our children that this is ok, and it isn't. We're showing them that it's ok to take substances to overcome the pain instead of focusing on the situation, talking about it, and resolving it. Subduing our emotions and feelings to help us deal with trauma then takes us away from being effective and close with our family members, so it's important to overcome this. When we learn how to do this from a young age, it is a behaviour that we can use for the rest of our lives, and gets passed down from generation to generation. It also means that we're developing who we are as people and growing to the next level, stepping into our power.

Don't get me wrong. It's all too common to take substances to alleviate the pain. This is actually what society subtly encourages us to do, with examples of celebrities like Amy Winehouse, Elton John, Michael Jackson, and Whitney Houston all abusing drugs and/or alcohol to cope with mental anguish. So how do we stop? We can't do it on our own, as we'll find ourselves going nowhere. There is plenty of research that tells us that when young people were exposed to talking therapies for example, they had fewer depressive symptoms than teens who had no treatment whatsoever. When we're holding onto our own stuff and not resolving it, it stays inside our minds and seems to grow into something else, a bitterness, resentfulness, and fear that we can't even see in our lives.

We were supporting a mentee and her family, Jessie had just turned 16 years old, had finished taking her GCSEs, and was about to go into the sixth form. Her family had noticed that her behaviour had changed and that she was more distant from them, spending more time in her room and on the Internet.

After being supported by a mentor, Jessie explained that she had gone to a graduation boat party to celebrate with the rest of the year 11s and drank a little too much alcohol. Because of that, when a boy asked for them to go to a quiet area to talk, Jessie agreed. He forced her to have sex and Jessie, overcome with alcohol, passed out. When she recovered – and she wasn't sure how much later – she was alone. She pulled her clothing together and returned to the boat party, keeping what had happened to herself. As a result, she was blaming herself for what happened and the fact that she had drunk too much.

Jessie's low opinion of herself reflected itself on her mood meter, where she ranked as in a state of high anxiety. Through guidance, she was able to see that because of drinking alcohol, she had been unable to make good decisions, and that in the future, she should not drink at all so she can make decisions with a clear head. We were also able to support Jessie in speaking with her family about this to enable all parties to accept that they weren't to blame.

Now Jessie has started university and is doing well, and the family has dealt with this situation and been there for their daughter. But can you imagine, however, if Jessie hadn't said anything and had continued to live her life? What decision would she have made about herself, with something like this happening to her when she was so young? What decision would she have made about men? What impact would this have had on Jessie and her future relationships? This is an example of some of the incidents that happen to us that as adults we don't talk about, that we don't resolve, and over which we end up taking substances to help us deal with the pain. Then, the longer we leave this incident unresolved, the more grip it has in our lives, even though its impact is invisible to us. One outcome as I have seen happen is that a woman who has experienced trauma as a child or young adult makes a decision about herself and a decision about men. But how does this work when she has children? How does she behave when her son is growing into a young man? Does she realise the way she's treating him is based on a decision she has made from her past that isn't resolved?

It is my reckoning that if there is an addiction to something, then you must look in the past for a trauma that you have experienced and not had support with. For you to grow emotionally, it is good if you can take that out of the closet and deal with it. It happened when it happened and the threat that was there then isn't there now. Because the actual threat has gone, we're left with our memories, which can be so painful that we feel like the trauma is still happening. We must be patient and allow those memories to heal and forgive yourself because in doing this you can heal and begin to move forward without the painful memories holding you back. Things are happening to us all of the time, and it is our choice whether we wish to hold onto them and give them power to influence our lives in the present, or whether we forgive ourselves, forgive the other person, and be in the now with our family members and give them our full love free from bitterness, sadness, regret, or upset. After all, what did they do to deserve that? And don't they deserve the best version of you that you can be? Also, living as a victim is no fun. It's tiring trying to behave as though nothing happened when something very big did. We go through all our lives like this, and this takes a lot of energy to put up this pretense.

Being a victim is hard work and it takes a lot of energy. We usually choose distraction to stop us from dealing with it (such as shopping, eating, drinking, or taking drugs, for example), and that is not who we really are. Furthermore, when we're being this way, the falseness of it all is being modelled to our children. Wherever we are a victim, there's a loss of power. Reclaiming that power can give us a feeling of peace like we've never had, with no need for substances to help us cope. But how can we deal with this in a way that moves us forward, giving us more peace and happiness in our lives and the lives of our family?

There are many things we can do, and here, I will look at the things that I have seen cause great transformations in people and their lives. Things that can really make a difference in our lives other than the things that we've spoken about so far. Many of our decisions in life are made because we draw from our own knowledge, belief, and understanding. Because we make many decisions from this place, we can be limited sometimes and we keep on doing the same thing, expecting the results to be different. For example, we can tell our child in a fit of anger that they're good for nothing and won't come to anything thinking that this would propel them into action. However, if we continue doing this, then that young person will believe it is the truth and take your words to be the beliefs they have about themselves. But what if, for example, you have an unresolved incident in your life, a rape, a sexual or physical assault, that you haven't resolved in yourself. Furthermore, what if you made a decision from that moment on that 'all men are rubbish', or that 'men only want one thing', or 'men are only good for one thing', or 'men cannot be trusted'. Your son will see exactly what you think of men through your behaviour and mannerisms. After all, when you made the decision, you didn't think to say, 'except my children', after all, boys and men are the same, you would consider them a threat. Now you can't see that in yourself, it's a blind spot. How can we find out about ourselves if we can't see it? Looking at the behaviour of others around us is a key as they will always reflect our behaviour. If we're still having difficulties in our relationship with our children, it may be because of something we can't see as it's in our blind spot. Have you ever been able to clearly see a fault or behaviour in someone else's life and wonder why they can't see it themselves? That's because you can see things more objectively, but they can't because it is in their blind spot. In the same way that you can see blind spots in your friends and family members, you have them too. However, have you ever tried to tell your friend or family members about themselves and their behaviour? Have you found that they listen? I would advise you not to say anything to anyone unless they ask you to tell them what you think. Normally, if people don't see their own blind spots, they don't see the solutions and the way through to resolve that area of their life. For example, with Jessie, she started blaming herself (a place of no power and blame), but changed to seeing that in the future, she would watch what she drinks as this would influence her to make unwise decisions (a place of power and responsibility). This is something that would have been in her blind spot had she not told anyone else about what she had been through and kept it inside for years.

We've looked at the impact of blaming our children and others for things that are happening in our lives. We know that this way of thinking is disempowering and restrictive. As a way of giving us power, we can see the answers in the behaviours of others and adopt ways and attitudes that enable us to grow emotionally. Also, seeing the impact of keeping things in our lives unresolved, the last thing to discuss here (and certainly not the least) is that if you have a tendency to blame others for your life, and why not, as it gets us off the hook of being the author in our own lives, it's probably likely that you're blaming God as well. After all, if we blame God for our situation, that means that we stay stuck in the same position and we don't progress. Why would we be blaming God for something? When a tragedy happens in our lives, a bereavement, an accident, when we have no control, we blame God. After all, it's His fault isn't it? However, this would be like blaming a friend that you haven't seen or contacted since you were kids. How can you blame your friend if you have no relationship with them? In a similar way, how can you blame God for something if you have no relationship with Him and you don't understand Him? Again here, blaming God is a great way not to progress in our own lives as we put the blame firmly at His door with an impact of becoming bitter and twisted as we deal with the consequences of our actions and behaviour. Today, we're in a blame culture, governments blame other parties and governments for things that are happening, divorcing parents are blaming each other for their behaviour and people are blaming teachers and schools for the knowledge and education of our children. We do this, as its easier to look at what's missing in someone or something else. However, this isn't the type of thinking that will forward the conversation and give us the emotional growth that we want and need to be those models to our children, that legacy that they will pass down to future generations.

In the next chapter we will look more deeply into ways that we can maintain the actions and behaviours we have put in place, to continue to grow and develop, giving you the life that you had said you wanted in the first chapter.

CHAPTER 7
Keeping your word

'You are what you do, not what you say you'll do'.
C. G. Jung

We have taken the first courageous steps in improving our child's emotional intelligence and used our child's behaviour as a reflection of what has been missing and supply what's needed to improve our relationship. In this chapter, we're going to take things one step further and look at ways of reclaiming the power that we've always had and, inadvertently, given away. Now that we have looked at the rules that you and your family can put in place, the next step is to apply each rule consistently, allowing rewards and sanctions/punishments.

Using reward and sanction charts

There are plenty of rewards and sanctions charts on websites like www.empoweringparents.com, among others. You'll find charts that you can modify and apply to your own circumstances and life, including charts for doing homework, household chores, and morning sequencing to get ready for school so your child learns through repetition each day. The objective of these charts is that ultimately, your child will learn to do what is needed of them without prompting or reminding. Put them up in your kitchen or public area and tick them off with your children. See their joy and sense of accomplishment when they see the good progress they have made. Also, similarly, listen to them when they don't follow their charts and find out why. At the same time, be consistent with the punishments for not following your instructions.

It is also important to think of sanctions and praises and stick to them also. I have taught many young people, and have seen the impact of some of the punishment and rewards they have had. One young man, 14-year-old Stevie, was doing very well in my lessons. He had started in my class and was disruptive. This was hiding a lack of belief in himself that he could do well in science. Fast forward one term, and he came first in his exams and he continued to do well. His poor behaviour had transformed into an interest and engagement. I gave him a letter praising him for the work he had done and proudly, he took it home and showed his parents. The next lesson, he returned beaming from ear to ear! 'Miss, miss, thank you for your letter, my parents couldn't believe that I had improved so much, they've paid for us to go to Florida this summer. I've always wanted to go there!'

This is an example of a reward that really made a difference! Maybe you can't afford family holidays to Florida, but there's always some type of reward to use as a form of acknowledgement or praise. I have seen parents treat their son or daughter to an event that they want to go to, a football match, going out for the day to the beach, as well as spending 15 minutes playing with them, or spending an afternoon having fun with them, finding more about their dreams for their futures.

Alternatively, for sanctions, there have been a variety of them that I've seen and the ones that are most effective are the ones where parents take things away and ground the child: taking away their phones (if they have phones), removing access to computers, and not allowing them to go out and socialize with their friends for a week or two. When parents have put these types of sanctions in place, I have seen a marked change in the young person, as they work hard to re-establish trust (and get their stuff back). There are other types of sanctions that aren't effective and that are physically and mentally harmful, such as screaming at or hitting the child.

Whatever sanctions and rewards you put in place, consistency is the key. You're showing your children what is reflected in the world, that good work is rewarded and breaking rules comes with punishment. In showing them this, it is more likely when they're adults that they will regard the rules, not break them in the first place, or if they do break them, then at least they won't try to get away with the punishments and fines put into place. We all know that trying to avoid paying fines in society just doesn't work as we always have to pay more in the end.

You can find examples of some sanctions that are tried and tested on www.empoweringparents.com. You know your child well enough to know what they will respond to.

I can't over-emphasize the importance of consistency. There were times when as a teacher I didn't want to apply a sanction and I did it anyway, and other times when I didn't apply the sanction, and looking back, I wish I had. It is all a learning curve. When I stepped over an incident, the young person thought that they can get away with something else, so sooner or later, I had to apply a sanction and speak with them about the impact of their behaviour. The impact of poor behaviour is an important place to look when applying sanctions. If a young person misbehaves, it wouldn't work to blame them for their behaviour, as this reduces their self-esteem and they continue behaving the same way to get negative attention in the belief that this is the only way that they can receive it. When a young person misbehaves, we must always look at the impact of their behaviour, what has happened as a result of their misbehaviour, because this focus is what develops their emotional intelligence and also their sense of responsibility, critical qualities for success in their lives, now and in their future.

One of our young people, 12-year-old Jenny, was excluded from school for fighting. She refused to interact with anyone and stayed in her room watching movies, for which she had a great passion. She would regularly disrupt her household by running out of the house without asking, resulting in the police bringing her back home in the small hours of the morning. Understandably, her parents were run ragged. This happened regularly every two or three weeks.

I started to support Jenny, showing her how to manage her moods. Jenny would regularly speak about how she was feeling and spoke about how she could change her mood or energy, especially if she was feeling low. I would invite her to look at the impact of her behaviour on her family, the lack of sleep, the worry, the concern, the disruption. This wasn't to blame Jenny, only her behaviour. When Jenny started evaluating her behaviour more, the times that she would cause disruptions became fewer and farther between. Eventually, Jenny started evaluating her behaviour without being asked to do so, and her family was happy because before we gave them our support, Jenny was not doing this. Jenny is now back in a comprehensive school after two years out of mainstream education, studying for her GCSEs, and continues to manage her moods every day.

Continue enforcing your rules, being consistent with sanctions and rewards for two weeks, and monitoring the changes each day in your journal. In addition, continue evaluating your mood and the mood of your child, and get used to speaking about your emotions to shift your energy and emotional state to your advantage.

Sticking to the plan

There are many times when I was teaching that I regularly evaluated myself and my behaviour and I learned that being consistent was the key. Never tell a child one thing, then do another. However, if we have to do that, we clean up the mess that we've made by looking at the impact. One time, I was carrying out a heart dissection with my year 8s – they were so excited! Due to a problem with our lamb hearts (the technicians couldn't defrost them in time for our lesson), I decided to postpone the heart dissection until the next lesson and focus on some theory of the heart to prepare the students. My students ran to my class all excited! 'Miss, miss, are we doing our heart dissection today?' To which I responded, 'I'm sorry, I've decided that it's best that we focus a little more on the structure of the heart today and do our dissection next lesson'. They weren't very impressed. One of the students replied, 'See how you are?' Well, I was surprised, to say the least! I always planned well and marked my lessons immediately after exams and homework as I found it fostered greater enjoyment and engagement, and this one time, this young student was pulling me up on what I had done! We say that 'talk is cheap' but really it's us that cheapens talk by saying and making promises and then not following through. When we do this with children, we're showing them that promises don't matter. We're also building up a distance between us emotionally, as they see that we're not someone they can count on. When you promise to do something for your child, you acknowledge that promise and you do what you said you would do. You don't decide not to do it because something came up and you weren't in the mood.

In this case, it is not about our mood, it's about being consistent. We wouldn't want our child to say, 'I'm not going to school today because I'm not in the mood'. When we look outside of ourselves and follow through on the promises we make to young people, we see that they look to us as someone who can be counted on, someone trustworthy. Also, we're modelling behaviour for them to follow as an example.

Planning reduces chaos

How can we stop reacting to circumstances and take control of them? All children like structure and discipline, and even if we say we don't, we all do. Doing nothing breeds boredom, which inhibits development and progress. Speak with your child and write down a plan. For example, if its football they love, then support them in joining the school football team and make sure that they're going every week. The same thing applies to you: Are you doing something that you enjoy on a weekly basis? Overlooking yourself doesn't work, as it means that you're not growing.

Sooner or later you'll get resentful, and when you operate from this emotion, your children will hook you easily. Before you know it, you're back to square one. Make sure you have a minimum of 15 minutes for yourself each day. Time alone for you to do what you really want to do, whatever it is, for example, praying, reading, walking, doing nothing, your favourite hobby, a mixture of all that has been mentioned. It is really important that you feed and strengthen yourself emotionally.

Make sure each one of you has at least one activity a week and place it on your calendar. I find an academic year-at-a-glance calendar works very well, as everyone can see it. Its A2 size, and you can even find them in the pound shops. Put it in a communal area like the kitchen area so everyone can see each other's schedule and know what's happening. Each family member can put their activities on the calendar. Most of these calendars have coloured stickers that you can colour code, one for each family member, if you like using them. Alternatively, write down the activities with a board pen (that comes with it) and make sure that everyone has a balance of activities. Also, make sure that you have the same amount of activities as your child. If they have one football or dance class once a week, make sure that you have something organised for yourself, also. Tick them off as you go through each week.

In the next chapter, we'll look at how we can maximise our wellbeing and health by putting simple structures in place.

CHAPTER 8
Onward and upward

'We ask ourselves, "Who am I to be brilliant, gorgeous, talented, fabulous?" Actually, who are you not to be? You are a child of God. Your playing small does not serve the world'.

Marianne Williamson

Putting It All Together

In this chapter we will look at all the things that could get in the way of achieving our goals and what we can do that will enable us to achieve our goals. We will look at how to strengthen ourselves physically, emotionally, and spiritually.

Emotional motivation

It can be relatively easy to engage in new behaviour when all is well. But when the going gets rough or we have a bad day, it's easy to revert to default behaviours, the old ones we got used to, and find ourselves back to square one. The good thing about these rough times is that there's a breakthrough around the corner, and we just need to get back onto that horse and keep going.

Having a goal or aim that really inspires you

What is your motivation for all of this? Why did you decide that this journey would be a good idea for you? Is it that you want to be a better role model for your children than you felt your parents were for you? Perhaps it's that you know that there's mental illness in your family and you wish to prepare your family with the tools they need to overcome it. Maybe you want to leave a legacy for your family for the following generations. You need to think of why you are doing this, write it down, and put it somewhere you can easily see it to remind you of why you are doing this. Believe me, you will have bad days and that's normal. It's important in these times to think of why you're doing this and the subsequent impact on your life and the lives of your children. Finally, does your purpose inspire you? The most important thing is that you inspire yourself.

Having friends that really inspire you

What about the network of friends you have around you? Do they inspire you? Can you relate to them? Or is it a one-sided conversation with them that relies on you to keep it going? This is something to take a look at with each friend and relationship. Check out the mood meter to see how they make you feel after you've been with them or after you've spoken with them. What we really want are friends that leave us in a positive mood, as these are the friends that will support us in those difficult times. Be careful of being around friends that leave you in a negative mood or even worse, in a negative mood and with negative energy (depression). That's not cool, and that's not the feeling and mood that you want to take to your family.

I would suggest decreasing the amount of contact with friends that give you a negative feeling and energy. You're not a dustbin, and these emotions will stop you from growing emotionally. I'm not saying that you tell them, 'I'm sorry, I don't want to have a friendship with you because you bring me down'.No, no, no, we need to be wise and prudent at all times. You will find yourself busy with other things and make your apologies, and in time they will find someone else to focus on.

Are you addicted to having these kind of relationships? Do you feel that supporting someone who drains your energy gives you more self-worth? Well you need to stop doing this, as it's not helping you and it's not helping them. They need to develop their own skills and grow emotionally, rather than dumping on you, and you have set your own goal to be a model for your children. It doesn't work for your children to see or be around this type of behaviour.

Having a partner that really inspires you

We haven't spoken much about your partner in this book, as it is essentially about you and your child. The two of you are modelling relationships for your child. So ask yourself, does your partner inspire you? What is it that is inspiring about them? Is there anything that's missing from them, in your opinion? Is it really them, or is it something about yourself? For example, if you think to yourself, 'They're not strict enough!', is it really that you're too strict? Have you spoken with each other so you have the same discipline strategy and beliefs? Are there any grey areas? If so, please get these all ironed out. Communication is the key here to loving and close relationships. When you speak with them about something that's missing, try not to blame them, after all, when you do that to anyone, they'll be backed into a corner and come out fighting, blaming you too! You look at yourself in that area, too, and talk about how this situation is occurring for you. Too often, we'll speak about something like it's the truth, when really it is just looking that way to us. If you find the two of you are seeing the same situation from two different perspectives, then this is worth discussing to help each other see the other's view point.

Physical motivation

Earlier in this book, we looked at the importance of mild exercise and healthy eating habits on our wellbeing and mood. Why should we continue this behaviour and how? Think back to the goal or objective you established that gave you emotional motivation, what was it? If you decided that you wanted to model important behaviour to enable your child to manage their moods and wellbeing forever, then an important part of this is managing physical health. For our systems to work well, we and our children need a minimum of 40 minutes to an hour of moderate physical exercise every day.

I know a family that transformed things for their child by buying him a massive trampoline. Every day after school, he would spend at least 30 to 40 minutes jumping on it. He found that it helped him eliminate the day's stresses, so he was able to be with his family and do his homework. What systems can you put in place that work for the whole of the family? Having playtime after school for the whole family has a great advantage for all to minimise the day's stresses. However, you must choose something that you like and enjoy, is it walking, cycling, running, hiking, dancing, roller skating, ice skating? Walking a pet? Find what you all enjoy and develop a routine.

This togetherness could also be incorporated as you develop your mealtimes, allowing your family to choose meals together and prepare them together. This may be a little difficult at first, but keep at it and increase the number of times a week you eat meals together. Young people love speaking about themselves, and quite often don't have an opportunity to talk. In the UK, parents are encouraged to work all hours to provide for their families, and sometimes don't have the energy nor the time to listen to their children.

When I was a teacher, I spoke with many young people who couldn't or wouldn't talk to their parents because they just didn't want to burden them or worry them. This is common. Young people often don't want to confide in their parents if they think their parents will find what they have to say upsetting, so they tend to keep things inside. We need to overcome this and let young people speak to help them find the answers to their difficulties and overcome their problems.

Spiritual motivation

What do I mean by spiritual motivation? I have spoken about the physical and emotional things you can do to transform your living situation and your lives to decrease the possibility of you and your child becoming stressed, anxious, or depressed. We have spoken about blame culture and that it's no wonder you were this way before. It's normal to blame everyone for our problems, including God. However, we now know that when we do this, we can't move on with our lives as we then judge that our lives are this way because of something or someone out there, nothing to do with us, and there is nothing, nothing at all that we can do about that.

The moment we look from a different perspective and see what we could have done differently, we see that we suddenly have new opportunities and pathways that we can take to achieve things we have only dreamed of in the past. We can stop making our lives into a soap opera, where we are the superhero and everyone else is the villain, and start looking at what we contribute to each of these situations.

It's also the same in our spiritual lives. We pray to God for something and wonder why we don't get it when we go around blaming everyone and Him for our lives. If you have suffered a tragedy, such as a death for example, blaming God may be your way of coping and surviving from day to day. However, this doesn't bring us happiness or joy. Anger simply gets in the way of dealing with our real feelings, those feelings that, when overcome, bring us to new actions and purpose in our lives.

I realised that I actually had turned my back on God way before I started experiencing challenging moments in my life. However, I thought it was that He turned his back on me. When I saw the truth, I felt a rush of relief travel through my body, a new hope for the future instead of feelings of bitterness, helplessness and regret. When we're in difficult situations and we don't know how we're going to get through them, we turn to things or people for support because that's what we're used to doing to get results. But sometimes alcohol or excessive shopping, just to give a couple examples, can't get us through those most difficult times, and for those times we need something more, something that's bigger and more powerful than the everyday people and things that support and guide us. Asking God for His support, guidance, strength, and power will help accelerate all of the things that you said you wanted family life to be like and more, facilitating a depth and love in your relationships and the closeness in your family.

How do you do this? There are two things you can do today that will make a marked difference. First, use five minutes of your 15 minute personal time (explained in the last chapter) to pray for all of the things you want to achieve, your dreams for your family, and yourself. Start with one or two minutes, thanking God for the things have you have, the things that are going well in your life. This can be your health or the health of your family, how your children are improving in school, just notice every little thing you can. Speak out loud as if you were speaking with your best friend. After you have thanked Him for all of those things you have and people that are around you, pray for what you need from him. For it to be an intelligent prayer (a prayer that God will listen to), you need to explain things in detail. Rather than saying, for example, 'Lord, I want to have lots of money,' try, 'Lord, I really do need more money because I would like to go to those book writing classes to develop my creativity, and when my children see that I'm studying it will really encourage them in their subjects at school too', or 'I would like to have more money so Jonny can go to those guitar classes and Jessica can go to her dancing lessons, because going to these lessons will help them develop themselves emotionally as well as increasing their development skills and I really want them to grow up to be well balance young adults'. Specific prayers and reflections like this will go a long way.

Do you have difficulty knowing exactly what to say? In that case, prepare a picture collage of how you would like things to be, finding photographs from magazines and the internet and sticking them into your note book. These could be pictures of a young person playing a guitar or dancing for example, if you would like Jonny and Jessica to go to guitar classes and dancing lessons. If you prefer to write, then keep a diary. The better clarity you have for your life and how it will look, the quicker God will answer your prayers.

Asking for strength will get you through those difficult days and time when you feel at your lowest. Be patient, Rome wasn't built in one day. You're building your home, and building it with patience, love, and commitment will enable you to build something that won't suddenly fall down.

The second thing you can do is open your bible (or Torah, or Quran) on any page and choose a verse (or two) and read it. When you're going through difficult times, find a verse in the bible that will lift you spiritually, giving you strength and power to continue your day, to change your mood and to give you (or restore) your hope. This needn't take long. Whatever verse you think you need to read, read that one, as that will be the Lord directing you. Think about that verse throughout the day, about what it means and how you can apply it to your life.

One parent, Sarah, told me that she was having a difficult time with her son, Mark, age four, who was really demanding of her time. She wasn't sleeping well, which was having a negative impact on her mood. She felt herself getting increasingly angry with every word and behaviour grating on her every nerve. One day, Sarah lost it and started criticising her son and shouting at him. Afterwards, she had regretted what she had done, and in her quiet moments of reflection and prayer, she opened up her bible, and saw that she was in Ephesians chapter 4. Her eyes drew her to verse 24, which said, 'Be angry and do not sin: do not let the sun go down on your wrath'. She knew immediately that this was guidance for her in her situation with her son, Mark. She read it, took in the message, and reflected for a few moments on what she needed to do, not to let the sun go down with her in this stage of anger and to apologise to her son, explaining that she didn't have much sleep and even though he was difficult sometimes that she would never do that again. Sarah asked Mark, 'Why do you behave like this? It makes me so mad and helpless and I don't know what to do to help you', to which Mark replied, 'Mummy, I like it when you do things with me and when I do good things, you don't know that I'm here'. From that moment, Sarah started talking with Mark in a way that they had never spoken. That day onwards their relationship changed. Sarah vowed that she would never shout and critique Mark again. Since that day, yes, there have been times when she feels angry, but what she read that day, 'do not sin', conveyed an important message to her to model good behaviour to her son.

In this chapter, we have looked at ways that we can maintain our new way of life and gain strength in times of weakness when we're wondering, 'Why oh why did I start doing all of this in the first place?' In times like these, look at the beginning of the book, where you wrote down how your life was and how you imagined your life could be. Compare your life now to how it was at the beginning and be thankful for all of the changes that have happened. In doing this, you will really see the progress that you have made, which in turn will give you room and space for further change. Also, acknowledge yourself for being the change that you are creating and for the great job you are doing.

CHAPTER 9
Obstacles

'We were born to make manifest the glory of God that is within us. It's not just in some of us; it's in everyone'.

Marianne Williamson

Back to Square One

So now you have changed your life over the last few weeks and really made a difference to your life and the life of your family. You've been making yourself accountable for your own moods and emotions and been the model for your children to increase their emotional intelligence. You've found parts of yourself, hidden jewels that were covered by fear, and by taking those first steps, you've seen parts of yourself that you love: your determination, your openness, and the resilience to make a big difference in your life and the life of your family. It's at times like this, when things appear to be going well, that sometimes we can make mistakes. We think, 'When I'm speaking more with my son, I'll be happy', or 'When I stop taking those tablets for depression, I'll be happy', 'When I start writing in my diary again, I'll be happy'.

Do not put your thoughts and dreams in the hands of someone or something else, as you'll be disappointed every time. You've started to take responsibility for every thought and emotion you have, and you've become able to shift your feelings depending on whether you want to feel more positive emotionally or whether you want to have more energy. Your emotions and moods are yours. You may not be able to control your circumstances, but you control your thoughts.

We all have 'off' days, and there will be days when you think everything is either all your fault or everyone's fault but yours. This is absolutely normal, but you're reading this book because being 'normal' doesn't work for you, you want to be exceptional.

Being exceptional and wanting an exceptional child means being an exceptional parent. And that means doing things that you didn't do before in the world of being 'normal'. Now, being exceptional is a whole different ball game. If you have stopped doing any of the new things that really have made a difference in your life, it doesn't mean that it's all over. Challenges are sent to test us, not to undo all of the hard work that we've taken on. Feeling guilty just stops you from really seeing the truth of what's happening, so forgive yourself and acknowledge yourself for doing such a great job. Keep on going because you will continue to reap the rewards with your new peaceful life. It may not all be now, but it will be soon, and lasting. You'll be surprised.

In my career as a teacher, I didn't realise that many years later, students would still be thanking me for how I contributed to their lives and their future, telling me how they have been inspired by me. Believe me, I wasn't thinking of this when I was in a new school, struggling to control my new classes! Sometimes I would say to myself, 'If you had let that student get away with that behaviour, you would have had an easier life'. However, I never let any behaviour slip past me, and I'm happy that I was like that, as now I see these young people being successful in their lives and I feel a pride when they speak with me and thank me. Did I know this would happen five years ago? No! However, it is one of the hidden benefits of sticking to my principles that I didn't even know was possible.

There are many things you could do that would stop your progress. You could start eating take-away food for a treat every now and then, which descends into chaos and eating badly again. Just get over it and move on, don't blame yourself and feel guilty, and don't say, 'I can't do this, it is too much!' because you have done it and you've overcome all of those obstacles.

If things start going wrong and you start going into blame, remember the main things: forgiveness, consistency, and being honest with your child about your mood and how you're feeling. You are building nothing less than their emotional intelligence.

Your goal through reading my book was to transform your relationship with your child. You wanted the support of this book to change things quickly. I want you to imagine that you have managed to solve your difficulties and that your dream of having that perfect relationship with your child has come true. How would you feel? How long do you think it would take?

I told my parents that they had done a good job with me when I was in my thirties. So you might have a while to wait before hearing these words from your child. But you can give yourself the gift of those feelings now. Write yourself a letter, from your child to yourself, dated 20 years from now. In this letter, thank yourself for doing a great job and teaching your child so well, for preparing him or her for the world out there. For helping them each day by modelling how you feel and how to change how you feel, for being consistent, for showing them how to enjoy preparing and being a connoisseur of food. What would you want to be thanked for and acknowledged for? What difference would you like to have made in the life of your child, and what tools would they find useful to be successful in their adult life? Whatever it is, it all starts here! It all starts now, sowing those seeds and making that difference, being that mum who was originally just a thought inside your head, and introducing her to the world.

CHAPTER 10
Back to the future

'As we are liberated from our own fear, our presence automatically liberates others'.

Marianne Williamson

So now you have changed you behaviour and put things in place to bring a newfound closeness between you and your child by talking and sharing mood states and what to do to change from one mood state to another. By now, you're speaking with more assuredness, more confidence, and greater knowledge of what works best for you and for your child. In addition, by changing your eating habits and your mealtime habits, you can further increase family cohesion.

What are the things you said you were committed to changing and transforming in your life at the beginning of this book? What is happening now? What changes have taken place? Keep on evaluating yourself, as it's important to acknowledge how far you've come. Keep on visualizing your child thanking your future self for being such a great parent and giving him or her the tools that they really needed and have used many times to help them make decisions and be the success that they are today. Take out that letter you've written and re-read it. It will happen, it's just a matter of time. It could be that when they are parents themselves, they will realise just how great you are and use many of your ways and strategies in their own parenting. Well done for starting something, starting with transforming yourself and the way that you deal with situations around you, leaving a legacy that will be passed down to your future generations, a legacy that will enable your children to be successful in their current and future personal and work relationships.

Congratulations for transforming your life!

ABOUT THE AUTHOR

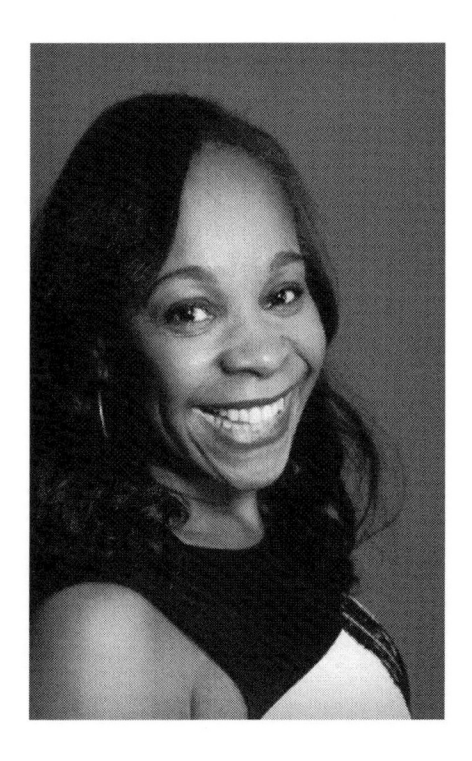

Jacqueline Campbell is the founder of the Julian Campbell Foundation, a charity that has made a difference to many young people, teenagers, and their families. The strategies used enable young people to identify and monitor their moods and develop their emotional intelligence.

With higher degrees in Education and Public health, Jaqueline began her career as a science teacher and went on to enjoy 20 years of teaching in some of the most difficult inner-city London schools, as well as training teachers.

From her time teaching in these difficult schools, Jacqueline saw that there was a need to support young people and their families to manage their wellbeing. For this, the Julian Campbell Foundation provides hands-on support to families through the training of mentors, trains teachers to identify young people who are exhibiting mild forms of mental health difficulty. The foundation also conducts drama workshops in schools, which provides a fun and light-hearted way to send an important lesson and message to young children, showing them how to identify and manage stress, anxiety, and depression in themselves and others.

Website: www.juliancampbellfoundation.org
Email: juliancampbellfoundation@gmail.com
Instagram: juliancampbellfoundation
Facebook: Jacqui Campbell/ Julian Campbell Foundation
Twitter: JulianCampbellF
LinkedIn: Jacqueline Campbell

THANK YOU

Thank you for reading *Runs in the Family*. The fact that you have got to this point in the book tells me something really important about you: You're ready to shift out of overwhelm. You're ready to experience clarity and peace of mind in your life.

This isn't the end, but rather the beginning of a new life and enjoyable future.

If you enjoyed this book, please write a review. I can always be reached through my website at www.juliancampbellfoundation.org or by email at Jacqueline@juliancampbellfoundation.org.

The income from this book will be donated to supporting young people overcome mental health difficulties so it can be given back to the community.

If you are ready to dive deeper and are interested in finding out more about Julian Campbell Foundation and our activities, we're offering *free introductory online videos* to all readers of our book. To have access to our free videos, please visit our online learning centre at www.juliancampbellfoundation.org.

Jacqueline Campbell

Printed in Great Britain
by Amazon